The Physician's Survival Guide to the Business of Medicine

Robert W. Katz, MS, CPA
Katz & Asher, LTD
New Orleans, Louisiana

AN ASPEN PUBLICATION®
Aspen Publishers, Inc.
Gaithersburg, Maryland
1994

Library of Congress Cataloging-in-Publication Data

Katz, Robert W.
The physician's survival guide to business of medicine / Robert W. Katz.
p. cm.
Includes bibliographical references and index.
ISBN 0-8342-0532-7
1. Medicine—Practice. I. Title.
[DNLM: 1. Practice Management, Medical—organization & administration—United States. W 80 K23p 1994]
R728.K38 1994
610/.68—dc20
DNLM/DLC
for Library of Congress
93-33907
CIP

Editorial Resources: Lenda Hill

Library of Congress Catalog Card Number: 93-33907
ISBN: 0-8342-0532-7

Printed in the United States of America

1 2 3 4 5

This book is dedicated to my beautiful and loving wife Jamie, without whose support it could not have been written . . .

to my darling daughter Stephanie . . .

to my mother, who instilled a love of reading and writing in me at a young age, and . . .

to Jesus Christ my perspective.

Table of Contents

Acknowledgments

I could not have written this book without the aid of several individuals who were at first clients. Over the years, however, I have become fortunate enough to count them as good friends. The editing and valuable insights offered by Austin Sandrock, MD, Hunter Watts, MD, Vicky Hebert, MD, Gerry Schneider, MD, Merrel Olesen, MD, Neil Baum, MD, and Jean Cukier, MD, have contributed immeasurably to this book.

I would also like to thank the following institutions and businesses for granting me permission to reproduce certain of their works: Practitioners Publishing Company, USAA's *Aide Magazine*, the USAA Foundation, A.G. Edwards & Sons, Inc, Zondervan Corporation, Bornstein Design Group, Halsey Publishing Company, and Delta Airlines.

Finally, I would like to thank the finest people with whom I have ever had the pleasure of working: the staff of Katz & Asher, Ltd, in particular my lifelong friend and partner Harold Asher for his patience throughout this project, and Rae Lynn LeBlanc, Karen Pistorius, and Linda Easterlin for their contributions. I could not have written this book without your help, support, and encouragement. It has been an honor to work with all of you.

INSERT

TAB

Introduction

Help Wanted

Job requires completion of years of expensive graduate studies and exhaustive on-the-job training. Customer expectations include that you be infallible. Should you fail, lawyers will point out the error of your ways. Federal and state agencies impose upon you an incredible assortment of rules, regulations, and paperwork and require you to provide more services for lower fees. Insurance companies, health maintenance organizations, and preferred provider organizations constantly question your charges, pay slowly, and second-guess your practice methods.

Sound like a great job? Then become a physician.

As a practicing CPA for 17 years, with many of those years spent traveling the country providing accounting and consulting services to physicians, it is obvious to me that being a physician is extraordinarily difficult.

Things are not going to get easier for physicians. Medicine is changing rapidly, and these changes will affect most physicians unfavorably, adding more stress and complexity to their lives. In the past, a mismanaged medical practice could do well in spite of itself. Soon, perhaps sooner than you think, only those practices that know how to operate as efficient businesses will survive.

◆ MEDICAL PRACTICE MANAGEMENT TRUTH 1 ◆

To enjoy future financial success, physicians must understand more than practicing medicine. They must understand the business of medicine.

This book, written especially for physicians, will show you how to survive, even in the most competitive environment. I guarantee, without hesitation, that if you follow just one of my recommendations you will recoup the cost of this book—probably tenfold. In my work with hundreds of physicians and their practices, I have learned which business methods work for physicians and which do not. In this book, I share this knowledge with you.

I find that most physicians fall prey to the same mistakes, which end up costing them tens of thousands of dollars and more. These mistakes fall into eight broad areas. This book is a practical approach on how to transform these eight potentially disastrous areas into eight areas of profitability:

- Using financial statements to manage your practice efficiently
- Properly setting and coding fees for services rendered
- Accounts receivable management
- Medical practice marketing
- Staff management
- Dealing with advisors
- Retirement planning
- Personal financial management.

The principles I recommend that you follow are not complicated. Implementing them in your practice will not be time consuming. Basically, the principles involve teaching you when, where, and how to look for problems and how to respond based on what you discover.

Many physicians with whom I work, caught in the midst of rapid changes, realize something is wrong with their practice, but they can't figure out what it is. Physicians are used to being organized, independent, and in control, so this kind of frustration is hard to handle. I see physicians throwing up their hands in despair and asking, "Why can't I just practice medicine anymore?"

There may have been a time when physicians could just practice medicine and earn a good living, but those days are gone forever. Let me repeat that. Those days are gone forever. The future will bring more demands from the public, lawmakers, hospitals, and corporations trying to carve out their share of the lucrative medical marketplace.

But don't despair. I wrote this book for the physician who wants to "just practice medicine." If you follow these instructions, I can assure you that your practice will be efficiently managed, leaving you as free as possible to just practice medicine.

Accountants are familiar with the story of the hot air balloonist who was blown far off course. He landed in a field, totally lost, and spotted a man walking nearby.

"Where am I?" he yelled.

The man replied, "You're in the basket of a hot air balloon in the middle of the field."

The balloonist shouted back, "You must be a CPA."

The man stopped suddenly. "How did you know?"

"It was easy to figure out," the balloonist said. "Your answer to my question was precise . . . and totally useless."

I've kept the lesson of this story in mind as I wrote this book. All the information is concise, practical, and useful.

◆ MEDICAL PRACTICE MANAGEMENT TRUTH 2 ◆

Ultimately, all your business and personal financial concerns will fall into one of three areas:

1. **your medical practice**
2. **your retirement plan**
3. **your personal financial situation**

Therefore, the book is divided into three sections. The eight areas of profitability I mentioned fall neatly into these three areas. Part I deals with your medical practice. Once you have completed this section, you will be able to see your practice as a constantly evolving business. You will learn to analyze your practice's health, at any point in time, so that you can quickly identify and solve problems. Most important, you will be able to set practice goals and easily monitor them so that, ultimately, you have an efficient, pleasant, and profitable operation.

Part II deals with your pension plan, or the pension plan you should have. This area of profitability has its own section because it is an often neglected yet vitally important part of a physician's financial well-being.

Part III deals with the basics of how to organize and analyze your personal finances. It also will encourage you to apply the same basic financial principles you now use in your practice to your personal finances.

If you learn how to control these three financial areas and understand how they interrelate, rest assured that you will have an efficient practice and sound personal finances for the rest of your life. It is just that simple.

INSERT

TAB

◆ Part I ◆

The Medical Practice

◆ Chapter 1 ◆

The Financial Statements Short Course

LESSON 1–1: ABSOLUTELY, POSITIVELY THE MOST IMPORTANT MANAGEMENT TOOL

An airline pilot, after several years of training and hard work, had finally attained his life-long dream: piloting the jumbo jets. As he got into his plush captain's chair on his first day at his new job, he couldn't help but be impressed by the complexity of the cockpit. As he guided the plane down the runway and into its take-off, he knew that he had truly become the master of high technology.

Unfortunately, a few hours after take-off his plane was struck by lightning. In a somber tone the pilot told his passengers, "I have some good news and some bad news. The bad news is that we have been struck by lightning. Communications have been knocked out. Fuel is running low, our guidance systems aren't working, and we are hopelessly lost."

The passengers waited.

"The good news is that there is a strong tail wind and we are making great time."

Every time I begin a new consulting engagement with a medical practice, this story comes to mind.

Physicians work very hard. So often in my work I encounter an extremely well-trained, hard-working group of physicians laboring at a feverish pace. Yet, like the pilot, many times they have no idea where they are headed. Eventually, lightning strikes. Fuel (cash) runs low, communications break down, and they get that same hopelessly lost feeling that the pilot had.

The good news for physicians is that in almost every case problems can be corrected before the practice crashes. Chapter 1 and its seven lessons lay the foundation for excellence in practice management. I say this because,

◆ **MEDICAL PRACTICE MANAGEMENT TRUTH 3** ◆

Without a doubt, your single most important practice management tool is properly prepared and analyzed financial statements.

Practice management begins with your financial statements. Unfortunately, many physicians find financial statements confusing and have little desire to learn to decipher their meaning. The beautifully bound booklet of financial statements is banished to a desk drawer or to the bottom of a stack of useless papers.

That's a shame. The truth is that financial statements are natural tools for physicians because you can and should approach them in the exact same manner that you approach your patients: diagnose and then treat. Properly prepared financial statements are your practice's periodic history and physical. By learning a few basic principles, you will be able easily to establish the health of your practice, diagnose its problems, and prescribe a treatment plan.

The remaining lessons in this chapter will teach you how to make your practice's financial statements the single most important diagnostic tool for practice management. Each lesson is based on one of six easy to understand and apply rules.

By the time you have completed Chapter 1 you will be an expert in analyzing financial statements. Using them, you will efficiently manage your practice.

The Golden Rules of medical practice financial statements:

- Financial statements *must* be customized for your specialty.
- Financial statements *must* be timely and accurate.
- Financial statements *must* be analyzed.
- Weaknesses in practice results *must* be isolated.

- Goals to correct weaknesses *must* be established.
- Practice results *must* be continually monitored.

As you begin to learn and apply these six rules, that hopelessly lost feeling will quickly begin to disappear.

LESSON 1–2: GOOD SUITS AND FINANCIAL STATEMENTS MUST BE TAILOR MADE

Medical practices are unique.

Medical practices are not usually capital intensive. They do not require a great deal of heavy equipment or a large investment in inventory. They are highly personalized, however, and quite often they deal in life-and-death issues.

Because they are unique, it is not acceptable for your accountant to use the chart of accounts for a retail store or for a restaurant and slap the name of your practice on top of it. This is often exactly how financial statements for medical practices are prepared. It is very difficult to extract meaningful management information from these poorly prepared statements.

All too often, accountants will prepare financial statements that help them prepare tax returns. What you must insist on are financial statements that provide you with meaningful information for management purposes.

Luckily, you do not need to be an expert on designing financial statements any more than you need to know how to sew your own suits. You can look in the mirror and know if the suit you just bought needs additional tailoring. The purpose of this lesson is to teach you how to look at your practice's financial statements to ensure that they provide you with the key financial information you need.

To accomplish this, view your medical practice, for business purposes, as a conduit, a pipeline. Yes, a pipeline. Money goes into the pipeline at one end and comes out the other through one of two spigots. The first spigot is practice operating expenses. These are the expenses necessary to keep the doors to your medical practice open. The second spigot is physician compensation and fringe benefits. Excellent financial statements will clearly report how cash is flowing through the pipeline and also will aid you in directing out of which spigot it ultimately comes.

But first, the basics. Financial statements for a medical practice should be composed of two reports: the balance sheet and the income statement.

The Balance Sheet

The balance sheet consists solely of a listing of medical practice assets and liabilities at one particular point in time. A typical balance sheet for a medical practice is uncomplicated. Exhibit 1–1 is a sample of a tax basis balance sheet for a typical medical practice. As you can see, as of one particular point in time (December 31, 1994) this practice's assets are cash, medical equipment, furniture, fixtures, leasehold improvements, and the accumulated depreciation. Liabilities on the balance sheet are a bank loan, an accrued pension plan contribution, and payroll taxes due.

Exhibit 1–1 Tax Basis Balance Sheet

A.B. Jones, MD: A Professional Corporation
Statements of Assets, Liabilities, and Equity
Income Tax Basis
December 31, 1994

ASSETS	
CURRENT ASSETS	
Cash—operating account	$ 4,000
Cash—money market account	20,000
TOTAL CURRENT ASSETS	24,000
FIXED ASSETS	
Furniture and fixtures	17,000
Medical equipment	50,000
Leasehold improvements	38,000
	105,000
Accumulated depreciation	(55,000)
	50,000
TOTAL ASSETS	$ 74,000
LIABILITIES AND STOCKHOLDERS' EQUITY	
CURRENT LIABILITIES	
Pension contribution payable	$ 30,000
Current portion of long-term debt	12,000
Payroll taxes payable	1,500
TOTAL CURRENT LIABILITIES	43,500
LONG-TERM DEBT, net of current portion (10% secured by equipment, due December 31, 1994)	24,000
STOCKHOLDERS' EQUITY	
Common stock, $1 par value, 1000 shares authorized, issued, and outstanding	1,000
Retained earnings	5,500
	6,500
TOTAL LIABILITIES	$ 74,000

See accountant's compilation report, attached

The Income Statement

The income statement, to me, is by far the more important financial statement for management purposes. The income statement reports income collected and expenses paid during a period of time, usually a month or quarter. When you first engage your accountant, he or she should confer with you regarding the design of your financial statements. Some of the more pertinent questions that you should discuss with the accountant are as follows:

- What are the basic expense categories for medical practices in general and for your specialty?
- What is the most meaningful method of reporting practice income? Does the practice require that income be reported by individual physician productivity, by office location, by certain departments, by specialty, or by payer sources (such as private pay, Medicare, or health maintenance organizations)?
- Is your group a single-specialty or multi-specialty group?
- Are there expense categories unique to your practice that your group would like to create and track as separate line item expenses?
- Do any expenses need to be categorized in a special way, such as by physician, by department, by office location, or by specialty?
- Are financial results summarized by department required? (For instance, a group of surgeons may have its own ambulatory surgical facility. Properly prepared financial statements would include departments that separate the financial results of the surgical practice from the financial results of the surgery center.)
- Does the practice want compensation reported by physician?
- Are there any other nuances particular to your practice that you would like to see reflected in its financial statements?

The following examples illustrate income statements that have been customized to satisfy the specific requirements of four different medical specialties.

All the examples have common features. For instance, regardless of the specialty the income statement is always divided into three sections. The first section summarizes practice income. The second section details the practice's operating expenses. The final section details physician salaries and fringe benefits.

Another common element is that every expense also is reported as a percentage of income. As you read the remainder of Chapter 1, you will understand why I believe that this feature is mandatory. Finally, all income statements should compare the results of the current and year-to-date periods with the same information from the prior year.

Exhibit 1–2 is the income statement of a solo practitioner urologist. This straightforward income statement illustrates the three basic sections discussed above.

Exhibit 1–2 Income Statement, Solo Practitioner

A. B. Jones, MD (APMC)
Statements of Revenues and Expenses
Income Tax Basis
See accountant's compilation report, attached

	For the Period 10/01/92–12/31/92				For the Period 10/01/91–12/31/91			
	Current-Period Amount	Cur-Pd Ratio	Year-to-Date Amount	Y-T-D Ratio	Same-Pd-Lst-Yr Amount	Pd-LYr Ratio	Y-T-D-Lst-Yr Amount	YTD-LY Ratio
INCOME								
Professional fees	$81,381.74	100.06	$345,441.37	100.93	93,720.11	99.03	$401,429.00	99.55
Interest income	222.58	.27	411.85	.12	994.20	1.05	2,188.05	.54
Refunds	(275.28)	(.34)	(3,589.63)	(1.05)	(78.95)	(.08)	(354.10)	(.09)
Total income	$81,329.04	99.99	$342,263.59	100.00	$94,635.36	100.00	$403,262.95	100.00
OPERATING EXPENSES								
Answering service	$(2,586.82)	3.18	$684.65	.20	$209.95	.22	$996.25	.25
Auto expense	178.25	.22	1,062.91	.31	1,043.97	1.10	4,412.66	1.09
Bank charges	86.71	.11	832.62	.24	109.31	.12	546.52	.14
Casual labor	.00	.00	.00	.00	.00	.00	575.00	.14
Collection expense	34.26	.04	155.24	.05	56.17	.06	175.49	.04
Continuing education	.00	.00	295.00	.09	405.00	.43	505.00	.13
Contributions	225.00	.28	350.00	.10	150.00	.16	195.00	.05
Conventions & meetings	.00	.00	100.00	.03	250.00	.26	305.00	.08
Depreciation	697.50	.86	2,550.00	.75	2,200.00	2.32	4,300.00	1.07
Dues & subscriptions	1,805.00	2.22	2,742.11	.80	1,419.00	1.50	2,311.68	.57
Entertainment	531.45	.65	8,554.41	2.50	.00	.00	.00	.00
Insurance–general	3,838.15	4.72	28,103.26	8.21	977.70	1.03	18,535.81	4.60
Insurance–hospital/disabil	.00	.00	5,051.09	1.48	3,309.87	3.50	8,649.89	2.14
Insurance–term life	.00	.00	.00	.00	.00	.00	3,912.39	.97
Interest	.00	.00	.00	.00	.00	.00	305.90	.08
Legal & accounting	850.00	1.05	5,300.00	1.55	675.00	.71	4,275.00	1.06
Linen & uniforms	216.35	.27	249.06	.07	.00	.00	45.46	.01
Medical supplies	2,698.88	3.32	15,691.55	4.58	3,370.89	3.56	14,761.70	3.66
Miscellaneous	229.84	.28	4,831.62	1.41	2,955.47	3.12	9,599.26	2.38
Office supplies	1,531.21	1.88	4,820.42	1.41	3,278.34	3.46	7,724.10	1.92
Postage	325.54	.40	1,677.81	.49	515.44	.54	2,041.30	.51
Professional fees	1,715.00	2.11	3,969.91	1.16	.00	.00	.00	.00
Rent	4,823.85	5.93	19,412.90	5.67	4,847.23	5.12	19,238.23	4.77
Staff salaries	14,639.85	18.00	45,607.41	13.33	15,822.52	16.72	44,162.34	10.95
Taxes & licenses	345.46	.42	785.72	.23	.00	.00	1,373.00	.34
Taxes–income	.00	.00	.00	.00	.00	.00	5,873.00	1.46
Taxes–payroll	1,976.03	2.43	9,183.73	2.68	2,406.94	2.54	9,344.00	2.32
Travel	263.54	.32	2,269.29	.66	2,491.01	2.63	7,079.44	1.76
Telephone	1,806.39	2.22	9,284.30	2.71	2,018.31	2.13	8,280.67	2.05
Unemployment–state	.00	.00	567.02	.17	66.19	.07	211.51	.05
Unemployment–federal	.00	.00	138.58	.04	.00	.00	37.75	.01
Total expenses	$36,231.44	44.55	$174,270.61	50.92	$48,578.31	51.30	$179,773.35	44.60
Income before professional compensation & pension expense	$45,097.60	55.44	$167,992.98	49.08	$46,057.05	48.70	$223,489.60	55.40
Officer compensation	$94,174.87	115.79	$168,000.00	49.08	$157,500.00	166.43	$234,000.00	58.03
Total compensation & pension	$94,174.87	115.79	$168,000.00	49.08	$157,500.00	166.43	$234,000.00	58.03
Net income	$(49,077.27)	(60.35)	$(7.02)	.00	$(111,442.95)	(117.73)	$(10,510.40)	(2.63)

Exhibit 1–3 is the income statement of an eight-physician, two-office pediatric group. In this example the physicians required that income be analyzed by office and by certain providers. Section 1 was customized accordingly. Additionally, the physicians requested that certain expense categories such as biologics, outside laboratory charges, chart costs, director's fees, and the like be reported as separate line items in section 2. In section 3 you can see that they wished to report compensation by physician.

Exhibit 1–4 is the income statement of a new plastic surgery practice that wanted to track income by physician because compensation was based on productivity. The physicians also wanted certain expenses, such as film and film processing, identified separately. Exhibit 1–5 is the income statement for a multioffice obstetrics/gynecology group that wanted income tracked in some cases by payer and in some cases by ancillary services, such as laboratory and radiology.

Additionally, Figures 1–1 through 1–8 offer examples of graphs and charts that you may wish to have your CPA prepare as part of your routine management reporting package.

A good accountant will work with you to ensure that your financial statements are customized to produce meaningful information. This does not have to be a complicated, drawn-out process. By answering a few pertinent questions and working with your accountant, you should be able to develop financial reports that will become valuable management tools.

Exhibit 1–3 Income Statement, Group Practice, Two Offices

Physicians Pediatrics
Statements of Revenues and Expenses
Income Tax Basis
See accountant's compilation report, attached

	For the Period 10/01/92–12/31/92				For the Period 10/01/91–12/31/91			
	Current-Period Amount	Cur-Pd Ratio	Year-to-Date Amount	Y-T-D Ratio	Same-Pd-Lst-Yr Amount	Pd-LYr Ratio	Y-T-D-Lst-Yr Amount	YTD-LY Ratio
INCOME								
Office A-fees	$251,073.74	48.60	$1,041,682.20	49.78	$272,677.70	$55.86	$1,067,044.95	53.08
Office A-HMO 1	53,561.31	10.37	195,784.53	9.36	44,079.78	9.03	187,109.63	9.31
Office A-HMO 2	5,265.00	1.02	42,367.91	2.02	9,841.12	2.02	92,489.53	4.60
Office B-fees	140,570.65	27.21	532,935.90	25.47	90,462.31	18.53	364,539.74	18.13
Office B-HMO 1	66,935.64	12.96	275,988.13	13.19	68,847.99	14.10	297,569.67	14.80
Office B-HMO 2	1,192.07	.23	8,808.11	.42	2,064.32	.42	2,440.90	.12
Interest income	134.26	.03	694.77	.03	505.26	.10	1,583.84	.08
Refunds	(2,146.95)	(.42)	(5,489.52)	(.26)	(303.84)	(.06)	(2,492.72)	(.12)
Total income	$516,585.72	100.00	$2,092,772.03	100.01	$488,174.64	100.00	$2,010,285.54	100.00
GENERAL & ADMIN. EXPENSE								
Advertising	$3,414.30	.66	$10,618.70	.51	$2,305.75	.47	$10,289.60	.51
Auto expense	.00	.00	.00	.00	1,700.00	.35	1,700.00	.08
Bank charges	998.49	.19	4,253.69	.20	652.81	.13	2,507.24	.12
Business gifts	2,412.97	.47	4,407.48	.21	1,718.16	.35	2,705.34	.13
Casual labor	.00	.00	.00	.00	.00	.00	50.00	.00
Collection expense	26.96	.01	190.60	.01	7.91	.00	224.50	.01
Computer services	7,865.00	1.52	12,075.75	.58	1,351.95	.28	4,367.85	.22
Continuing education	.00	.00	1,985.00	.09	.00	.00	2,510.00	.12
Contributions	125.00	.02	625.00	.03	575.00	.12	1,151.00	.06
Depreciation	8,151.66	1.58	22,894.43	1.09	6,923.03	1.42	24,955.63	1.24
Directors fees	.00	.00	8,138.00	.39	.00	.00	.00	.00
Dues, subscription & books	8,149.65	1.58	13,541.44	.65	7,843.86	1.61	15,043.98	.75
Equipment rental	2,452.17	.47	9,380.30	.45	2,323.11	.48	7,818.09	.39
Insurance-general	38,796.00	7.51	44,468.00	2.12	34,419.00	7.05	39,034.00	1.94
Insurance-hospital/disability	39,001.30	7.55	77,376.16	3.70	12,103.92	2.48	45,219.03	2.25
Interest expense	.00	.00	2,581.49	.12	1,242.53	.25	8,594.36	.43
Janitorial	1,025.00	.20	3,725.00	.18	900.00	.18	3,650.00	.18
Laboratory	13,232.31	2.56	47,042.16	2.25	10,711.22	2.19	39,939.50	1.99
Medical supplies	5,935.44	1.15	25,725.50	1.23	4,270.38	.87	18,236.17	.91
Biologicals	58,480.72	11.32	270,705.57	12.94	31,109.93	6.37	197,611.82	9.83
Kitchen supplies	1,411.11	.27	4,232.60	.20	702.80	.14	2,169.94	.11
Office supplies	3,266.47	.63	10,645.91	.51	2,090.86	.43	6,438.82	.32
Office supplies-charts	1,589.65	.31	2,949.58	.14	488.94	.10	3,028.65	.15
Computer supplies	4,361.77	.84	8,889.14	.42	1,570.92	.32	6,589.95	.33
Postage	730.55	.14	8,494.92	.41	567.53	.12	4,973.74	.25
P C P-paps	.00	.00	.00	.00	.00	.00	4.08	.02
Practice promotion	2,849.10	.55	5,527.59	.26	.00	.00	.00	.00
Stationery & printing	483.18	.09	1,960.47	.09	190.22	.04	1,336.22	.07
Professional fees	7,948.79	1.54	31,455.44	1.50	6,243.04	1.28	29,423.90	1.46
Recruitment	.00	.00	4,789.76	.23	5,743.28	1.18	10.866.11	.54
Rent	29,090.25	5.63	116,361.00	5.56	29,090.25	5.96	101,167.50	5.03
Repairs & maintenance	3,588.94	.69	15,757.68	.75	10,306.10	2.11	27,570.69	1.37
Staff salaries	134,356.32	26.01	464,423.56	22.19	129,319.33	26.49	426,538.76	21.22
Storage	408.00	.08	1,608.00	.08	396.00	.08	1,559.00	.08
Taxes & licenses	2,447.29	.47	2,764.78	.13	3,242.46	.66	4,129.11	.21
Taxes-income	.00	.00	1,684.00	.08	.00	.00	.00	.00
Taxes-payroll	15,107.51	2.92	77,824.63	3.72	16,025.41	3.28	77,118.56	3.84
Telephone & telegraph	5,080.14	.98	21,703.48	1.04	6,244.02	1.28	26,625.19	1.32
Travel	140.00	.03	2,436.86	.12	.00	.00	944.15	.05
Unemployment-federal	117.12	.02	1,745.12	.08	198.57	.04	617.49	.03
Uniforms	.00	.00	185.01	.01	653.87	.13	1,582.50	.08
Total G & A expense	$403,043.16	77.99	$1,345,173.80	64.27	$333,232.16	68.24	$1,158,696.39	57.64
INCOME BEFORE PROFESSIONAL COMPENSATION & PENSION EXPENSE	$113,542.56	22.01	$747,598.23	35.74	$154,942.48	31.76	$851,589.15	42.36
Salary-Dr 1	$33,531.00	6.49	$110,720.26	5.29	$42,167.00	8.64	$126,064.00	6.27
Salary-Dr 2	.00	.00	9,200.00	.44	14,800.00	3.03	54,200.00	2.70
Salary-Dr 3	36,527.00	7.07	113,879.00	5.44	42,930.00	8.79	131,088.00	6.52
Salary-Dr 4	19,975.00	3.87	71,866.00	3.43	21,755.00	4.46	86,105.00	4.28
Salary-Dr 5	35,837.00	6.94	110,910.00	5.30	36,883.00	7.56	121,130.00	6.03
Salary-Dr 6	41,804.00	8.09	146,962.00	7.02	53,072.00	10.87	130,231.00	6.48
Salary-Dr 7	38,823.00	7.52	122,460.00	5.85	36,242.00	7.42	120,755.00	6.01
Salary-Dr 8	6,540.00	1.27	6,540.00	.31	.00	.00	.00	.00
Pension expense	82,873.04	16.04	82,873.04	3.96	.00	.00	.00	.00
Total compensation & pension	$295,910.04	57.29	$775,410.30	37.04	$247,849.00	50.77	$769,573.00	38.29
Net income	$(182,367.48)	(35.28)	$(27,812.07)	(1.30)	$(92,906.52)	(19.01)	$82,016.15	4.07

Exhibit 1–4 Income Statement, Group Practice

Plastic Surgery Associates
Statements of Revenues and Expenses
Income Tax Basis
See accountant's compilation report, attached

	For the Period 10/01/92–12/31/92				For the Period 10/01/91–12/31/91			
	Current-Period Amount	Cur-Pd Ratio	Year-to-Date Amount	Y-T-D Ratio	Same-Pd-Lst-Yr Amount	Pd-LYr Ratio	Y-T-D-Lst-Yr Amount	YTD-LY Ratio
INCOME								
Fees-Dr A	$98,643.14	65.49	$1,316,603.10	71.17	$131,567.93	78.52	$1,542,459.94	74.69
Fees-Dr B	200.00	.13	2,284.16	.12	225.00	.13	133,162.77	6.45
Fees-Dr C	26,794.50	17.79	261,073.80	14.11	10,932.66	6.52	232,104.91	11.24
Fees-Dr D	15,734.66	10.45	229,517.74	12.41	24,290.92	14.50	147,473.05	7.14
Fees-Dr E	.00	.00	10,910.00	.59	.00	.00	.00	.00
	1,944.00	1.29	9,530.68	.52	451.00	.27	6,408.60	.31
Skin care products income	1,530.00	1.02	4,566.17	.25	.00	.00	.00	.00
Miscellaneous income	5,780.98	3.84	15,458.29	.84	41.20	.02	3,590.30	.17
Patient refunds	.00	.00	.00	.00	50.00	.03	.00	.00
Total income	$150,627.28	100.01	$1,849,943.94	100.01	$167,558.71	99.99	$2,065,199.57	100.00
GENERAL & ADMINISTRATIVE								
Advertising	$20,045.67	13.31	$279,466.44	15.11	$27,365.37	16.33	$300,026.19	14.53
Auto expense	.00	.00	.00	.00	.00	.00	1,709.73	.08
Anesthesia supplies/gasses	.00	.00	127.00	.01	.00	.00	.00	.00
Bank charges	1,756.18	1.17	14,953.91	.81	1,856.49	1.11	9,711.41	.47
Casual labor	.00	.00	1,467.75	.08	.00	.00	276.25	.01
Computer expense	98.41	.07	12,006.59	.65	.00	.00	3,338.55	.16
Consultants	.00	.00	4,340.20	.23	500.00	.30	700.00	.03
Continuing education	(400.00)	(.27)	1,914.00	.10	400.00	.24	1,479.00	.07
Cosmetic services	2,811.76	1.87	7095.38	.38	.00	.00	440.00	.02
Depreciation/amortization	5,704.64	3.79	64,360.10	3.48	14,010.37	8.36	37,585.08	1.82
Drugs & pharmacy	100.00	.07	1,518.65	.08	220.00	.13	11,263.22	.55
Dues & subscriptions	47.80	.03	5,208.54	.28	1,918.80	1.15	6,816.22	.33
Equipment rental	179.49	.12	2,923.96	.16	209.49	.13	3,846.30	.19
Film & processing	596.38	.40	8,836.02	.48	(2,903.72)	(1.73)	9,010.26	.44
Insurance-general	390.00	.26	5,199.64	.28	438.00	.26	4,254.60	.21
Insurance-malpractice	.00	.00	.00	.00	.00	.00	5,404.00	.26
Insurance-hosp/disability	1,648.16	1.09	14,687.88	.79	1,129.40	.67	16,207.21	.78
Interest expense	887.18	.59	14,284.86	.77	1,325.00	.79	21,212.59	1.03
Laboratory	698.40	.46	3,182.75	.17	.00	.00	34.50	.00
Laundry/linen/uniforms	450.00	.30	5,301.88	.29	269.47	.16	4,400.98	.21
Legal & accounting	3,223.89	2.14	33,085.63	1.79	45,918.20	27.40	92,396.35	4.47
Medical supplies	.00	.00	10,516.50	.57	.00	.00	38,607.48	1.87
Miscellaneous	.00	.00	.00	.00	4,192.73	2.50	4,192.73	.20
Office supplies & equipment	2,347.93	1.56	29,801.00	1.61	12,021.17	7.17	48,371.62	2.34
Parking	510.00	.34	6,136.00	.33	510.00	.30	5,378.00	.26
Postage	288.54	.19	6,046.16	.33	808.12	.48	5,032.00	.24
Practice promotion	3,195.70	2.12	14,661.01	.79	415.12	.25	11,679.92	.57
Rent	12,285.75	8.16	144,593.82	7.82	11,813.22	7.05	122,699.38	5.94
Repairs & maintenance	3,415.77	2.27	31,617.87	1.71	2,161.36	1.29	36,179.12	1.75
Salaries-staff	30,295.19	20.11	313,026.46	16.92	14,390.62	8.59	224,065.43	10.85
Tax & licenses	160.00	.11	2,479.19	.13	.00	.00	615.00	.03
Taxes-income & franchise	6,000.00	3.98	48,045.00	2.60	.00	.00	896.00	.04
Taxes-payroll	2,182.68	1.45	31,325.48	1.69	345.28	.21	23,838.15	1.15
Telephone	1,470.55	.98	16,416.94	.89	529.43	.32	17,610.92	.85
Travel	1,101.33	.73	6,269.67	.34	2,762.42	1.65	4,217.03	.20
Utilities	312.32	.21	5,159.56	.28	55.61	.03	4,411.76	.21
Waste disposal	.00	.00	.00	.00	.00	.00	957.50	.05
Total expenses	$101,803.72	67.61	$1,146,055.84	61.95	$142,661.95	85.14	$1,078,864.48	52.21
Income before professional contracts	$48,823.56	32.40	$703,888.10	38.06	$24,896.76	14.85	$986,335.09	47.79
PROFESSIONAL CONTRACTS								
Contract-Dr A	$81,034.39	53.80	$502,630.93	27.17	$22,360.10	13.34	$577,311.92	27.95
Contract-Dr B	.00	.00	595.35	.03	101.25	.06	66,584.01	3.22
Contract-Dr c	12,113.02	8.04	122,233.31	6.61	4,949.70	2.95	111,249.38	5.39
Contract-Dr D	8,112.60	5.39	109,290.28	5.91	12,293.30	7.34	87,820.43	4.25
Contract-Dr E	.00	.00	.00	.00	.00	.00	445.00	.02
Contract-Dr F	.00	.00	2,911.50	.16	.00	.00	.00	.00
Total compensation	$101,260.01	67.23	$737,661.37	39.88	$39,704.35	23.69	$843,410.74	40.83
Net income (loss)	$(52,436.45)	(34.83)	$(33,773.27)	(1.82)	$(14,807.59)	(8.84)	$142,924.35	6.96

Exhibit 1–5 Income Statement, Group Practice, Multioffice

OB-GYN Associates
Statements of Revenues and Expenses
Income Tax Basis
See accountant's compilation report, attached

	For the Period 10/01/92–12/31/92				For the Period 10/01/91–12/31/91			
	Current-Period Amount	Cur-Pd Ratio	Year-to-Date Amount	Y-T-D Ratio	Same-Pd-Lst-Yr Amount	Pd-LYr Ratio	Y-T-D-Lst-Yr Amount	YTD-LY Ratio
INCOME								
Professional fees	$620,505.71	82.29	$2,432,024.42	80.95	$467,988.48	76.82	$2,358,509.57	79.39
HMO 1	58,830.48	7.80	226,982.56	7.56	67,042.12	11.00	259,709.15	8.74
Research income	.00	.00	5,010.00	.17	.00	.00	7,092.54	.24
Lab fees	66,412.35	8.81	296,432.07	9.87	68,787.00	11.29	307,966.00	10.37
X-ray fees	26,080.00	3.46	107,620.00	3.58	25,620.00	4.21	95,220.00	3.21
Miscellaneous income	.00	.00	.00	.00	.00	.00	8,942.58	.30
Interest income	1,666.67	.22	6,614.03	.22	3,123.10	.51	11,507.66	.39
Refunds	(19,483.67)	(2.58)	(70,379.64)	(2.34)	(23,354.98)	(3.83)	(78,193.53)	(2.63)
Total income	$754,011.54	100.00	$3,004,303.44	100.01	$609,205.72	100.00	$2,970,753.97	100.01
GENERAL & ADMIN. EXPENSE								
Bank charges	$419.97	.96	$2,176.50	.07	$269.95	.04	$1,065.99	.04
Business gifts	618.80	.08	1,436.47	.05	2,606.03	.43	3,187.74	.11
Casual labor	1,114.00	.15	3,138.18	.10	40.00	.01	1,675.56	.06
Collection expense	784.99	.10	2,609.44	.09	780.80	.13	4,356.12	.15
Computer services	1,070.69	.14	6,912.69	.23	2,244.38	.37	40,976.61	.37
Continuing education	(1,040.00)	(.14)	5,945.00	.20	1,564.00	.26	4,702.00	.16
Contributions	15.00	.00	15.00	.00	56.08	.01	65.11	.00
Conventions & meetings	.00	.00	.00	.00	140.00	.02	750.00	.03
Data processing fees	210.20	.03	1,319.65	.04	301.95	.05	1,375.00	.05
Depreciation	13,800.19	1.83	52,009.75	1.73	15,148.63	2.49	57,638.72	1.94
Directors fee	.00	.00	.00	.00	51,691.59	8.49	51,691.59	1.74
Donations	240.00	.03	2,630.00	.09	1,925.00	.32	6,502.50	.22
Dues & subscriptions	967.00	.13	8,357.01	.28	11,205.28	1.84	27,923.92	.94
Equipment rental	(331.70)	(.04)	(1,123.37)	(.04)	207.29	.03	1,447.30	.05
Insurance-general	85,420.00	11.33	90,431.00	3.01	68,287.00	11.21	73,018.00	2.46
Insurance-hospital/ disability	16,209.25	2.15	77,882.73	2.59	20,164.06	3.31	58,875.34	1.98
Insurance-term life	5,020.49	.67	28,670.08	.95	(4,035.07)	(.66)	15,201.75	.51
Interest expense	1,383.08	.18	11,106.00	.37	3,857.02	.63	19,132.34	.64
Laundry	580.00	.08	1,261.00	.04	190.50	.03	597.50	.02
Medical reimbursement	.00	.00	263.00	.01	1,042.92	.17	1,932.52	.07
Medical supplies	8,959.44	1.19	49,480.02	1.65	15,631.57	2.57	44,954.50	1.51
Miscellaneous	624.75	.08	2,126.72	.07	1,258.90	.21	5,010.03	.17
Office supplies	4,380.73	.58	39,124.18	1.30	6,857.17	1.13	27,584.32	.93
Misc-lab	.00	.00	.00	.00	.00	.00	29.00	.00
Postage	3,808.46	.51	15,181.28	.51	3,709.28	.61	14,030.42	.47
Pharmaceuticals	1,555.15	.21	3,906.16	.13	398.42	.07	1,573.21	.05
Practice promotion	884.71	.12	8,631.83	.29	3,849.36	.63	10,531.62	.35
Stationery & printing	745.01	.10	8,318.25	.28	1,781.86	.29	6,044.70	.20
Professional fees	4,850.51	.64	28,087.91	.93	4,485.00	.74	25,292.24	.85
Malpractice defense	2,579.80	.34	12,371.61	.41	17,876.46	2.93	37,047.50	1.25
Recruitment	(1,061.63)	(.14)	(521.68)	(.02)	195.48	.03	2,084.40	.07
Rent	24,133.45	3.20	116,991.55	3.89	33,289.32	5.46	133,559.91	4.50
Repairs & maintenance	2,908.91	.39	18,346.99	.61	17,797.18	2.92	39,832.03	1.34
Research expense	949.25	.13	4,515.25	.15	1,088.00	.18	6208.98	.21
Services	856.26	.11	3,968.78	.13	1,078.25	.18	4,305.50	.14
Salaries-staff	98,768.40	13.10	403,107.14	13.42	95,104.16	15.61	373,277.22	12.57
Salaries-administrator	16,049.30	2.13	62,495.66	2.08	15,472.34	2.54	59,952.42	2.02
Taxes & licenses	4,424.00	.59	6,574.00	.22	7,883.85	1.29	15,920.23	.54
Taxes-payroll	11,295.11	1.50	82,975.77	2.76	11,504.47	1.89	96,490.39	3.25
Telephone & telegraph	11,391.96	1.51	47,845.28	1.59	12,657.98	2.08	47,978.78	1.62
Travel & entertainment	7,732.21	1.03	28,371.55	.94	6,706.89	1.10	9,807.77	.33
Uniforms	901.83	.12	2,677.34	.09	1,140.67	.19	1,889.83	.06
Fertility studies	94.34	.01	363.03	.01	148.20	.02	1,626.71	.05
Linen-lab	264.25	.04	1,039.48	.03	291.97	.05	961.74	.03
Outside services-lab	6,572.43	.87	39,088.46	1.30	10,466.67	1.72	40,396.70	1.36
Printing-lab	.00	.00	117.23	.00	.00	.00	294.12	.01
Professional fees-lab	7,745.00	1.03	37,187.00	1.24	8,686.00	1.43	35,626.00	1.20
Professional fees-X-ray	.00	.00	109.64	.00	.00	.00	.00	.00
Rent-lab	2,101.26	.28	8,405.04	.28	2,101.26	.34	8,405.04	.28
Repairs & maintenance-lab	341.60	.05	3,468.35	.12	771.06	.13	1,437.15	.05
Salaries-lab	15,809.53	2.10	63,164.19	2.10	14,822.89	2.43	59,172.28	1.99
Supplies-office-lab	.00	.00	.00	.00	85.00	.01	580.23	.02
Supplies-scientific-lab	7,675.07	1.02	41,220.10	1.37	12,153.68	2.00	50,750.44	1.71
Supplies-X-ray	3,607.25	.48	12,614.51	.42	4,424.35	.73	14,763.10	.50
Total G & A expense	$377,430.30	50.10	$1,446,392.75	48.11	$491,405.10	80.69	$1,519,534.12	51.17
Income before Drs. comp.	$376,581.24	49.90	$1,557,910.69	51.90	$117,800.62	19.31	$1,451,219.85	48.84
PROFESSIONAL COMPENSATION								
Salary-Dr A	$84,964.37	11.27	$226,940.77	7.55	$73,731.42	12.10	$202,072.82	6.80
Salary-Dr B	85,084.56	11.28	261,299.76	8.70	73,184.56	12.01	235,199.76	7.92
Salary-Dr C	36,576.90	4.85	117,499.90	3.91	35,576.90	5.84	127,499.90	4.29
Salary-Dr D	79,730.76	10.57	233,699.96	7.78	64,230.76	10.54	217,199.96	7.31
Salary-Dr E	79,730.76	10.57	240,899.96	8.02	66,630.76	10.94	219,599.96	7.39
Salary-Dr F	.00	.00	.00	.00	.00	.00	34,285.75	1.15
Salary-Dr G	79,730.76	10.57	233,699.96	7.78	64,230.76	10.54	219,599.96	7.39
Profit sharing plan	148,227.47	19.66	198,227.47	6.60	19,025.34	3.12	194,025.34	6.53
Total compensation	$594,045.58	78.77	$1,512,267.78	50.34	$396,610.50	65.09	$1,449,483.45	48.78
Net income	$(217,464.34)	(28.87)	$45,642.91	1.56	$(278,809.88)	(45.78)	$1,736.40	.06

LESSON 1–3: IF THEY'RE NOT ON TIME AND ACCURATE, THROW 'EM BACK

Do any of these phrases sound familiar to you?

"I hardly ever see my accountant. I don't know how often he prepares financial statements for me. Once a year, I think, he uses them to prepare my tax returns."

"After the quarter ends, it's months before I get any financial statements."

"My financial statements come in the mail. My accountant never sits down and explains them to me. I don't even know why I need them. They just seem like a waste of money."

"They usually have a lot of mistakes in them, and the office manager winds up having to make several corrections to them."

If these statements describe your situation, it means that you have been abandoned and left to manage your practice in the dark. The result is what I refer to as checkbook management. This means that if there is money in your checkbook you feel OK. If there isn't, then you have a vague notion of a problem. The problem with checkbook management is that you are constantly treating symptoms. Checkbook management never allows you to focus on real practice problems until they are serious. Timely, accurate financial statements give you the information that you need to identify problem areas and react expeditiously before they become crises.

Here are the basic rules of performance that you should insist on from your accountant:

- Your practice's financial statements must be prepared at least quarterly.
- The financial statements must be in your hands no later than the last day of the month after the close of a period. For instance, for the quarter that ends June 30, you must have your financial statements by July 31.
- Your accountant should spend at least an hour reviewing the results with you.
- The statements must be accurate.

These rules certainly do not place onerous demands on your accountant. Obviously, no accountant will be perfect. Occasionally, statements may take a little longer than 30 days to prepare, and some errors are inevitable. If your accountant can't comply with the above guidelines at least 98% of the time, however, I strongly recommend that you terminate his or her services and find one who can. If you are to remain competitive, you must run your practice as a business, even if it means making unpleasant decisions.

What would happen if you took six weeks to give a patient a test result? Imagine the consequences if Exxon were to tell shareholders consistently, "Sorry, but our financial statements won't be ready for several months" or if they issued statements that were consistently full of errors? It would be impossible for them to manage their operation properly or plan for the future. Heads would roll. Your business is every bit as important to you as Exxon is to its shareholders. Therefore, the same foundation needs to be laid.

Timely, accurate financial statements used for management and planning will provide your practice with one of the competitive edges that it will need to succeed in tomorrow's marketplace.

LESSON 1–4: NUMBERS HARDLY EVER LIE

OK, you have in hand your custom-tailored financial statements that have been prepared in an accurate, timely manner. Practice management begins here.

We want to use financial statements to identify key factors. Key factors are critical operating results upon which the success or failure of your practice hinges. Each practice may have slightly different key factors. Examples of key factors from the financial statements might be practice collections, total practice expenses, physician income or revenue, and expense per case. You may wish to instruct your accountant to identify several key factors and to track them graphically for you. Figures 1–1 through 1–8 are graphs of key factors. We will discuss other key factors later in this book.

This lesson will instruct you on how to analyze these financial statements and how to identify your practice's strengths and weaknesses by means of key factor management:

- Identify the key factors for your practice.
- Develop expectations for those key factors.
- Identify areas of concern.
- Solve the problem.
- Repeat the process through continually monitoring key factors.

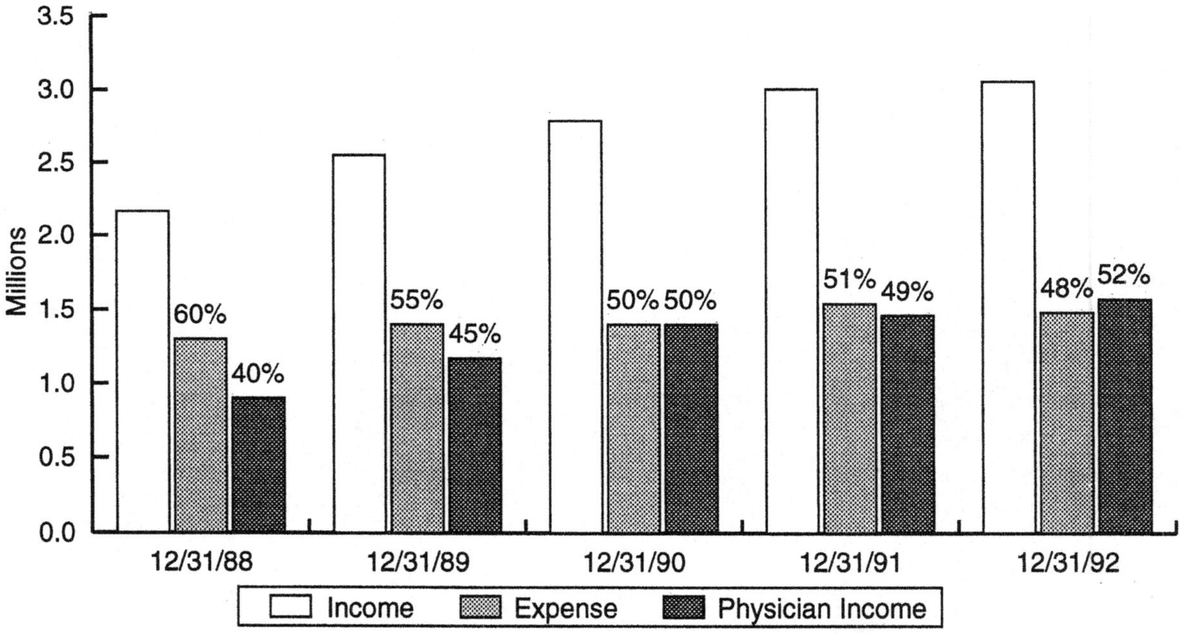

Figure 1–1 Analysis of gross practice income, expenses, and physician compensation.

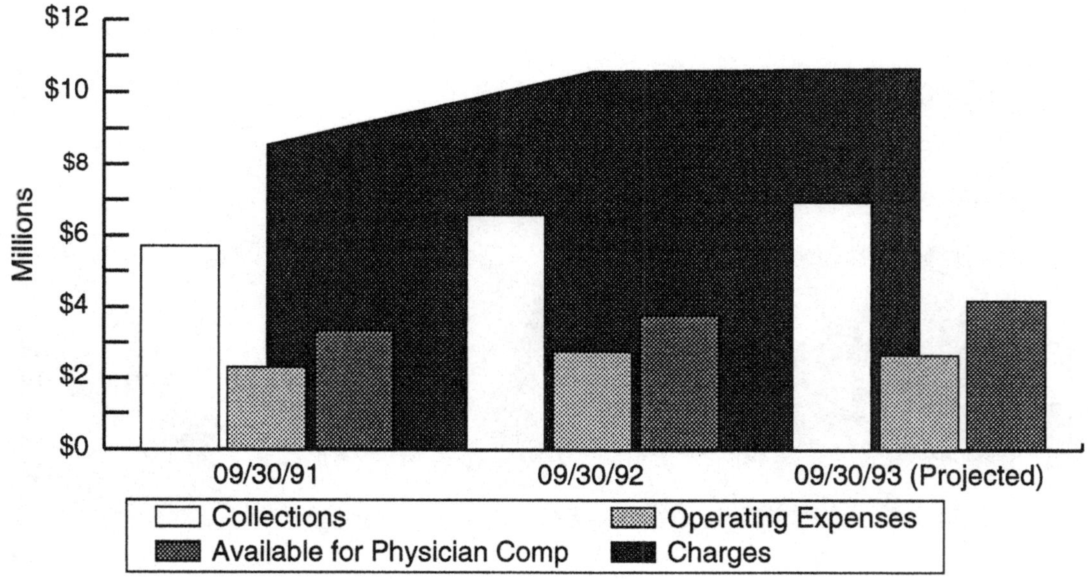

Figure 1–2 Performance analysis.

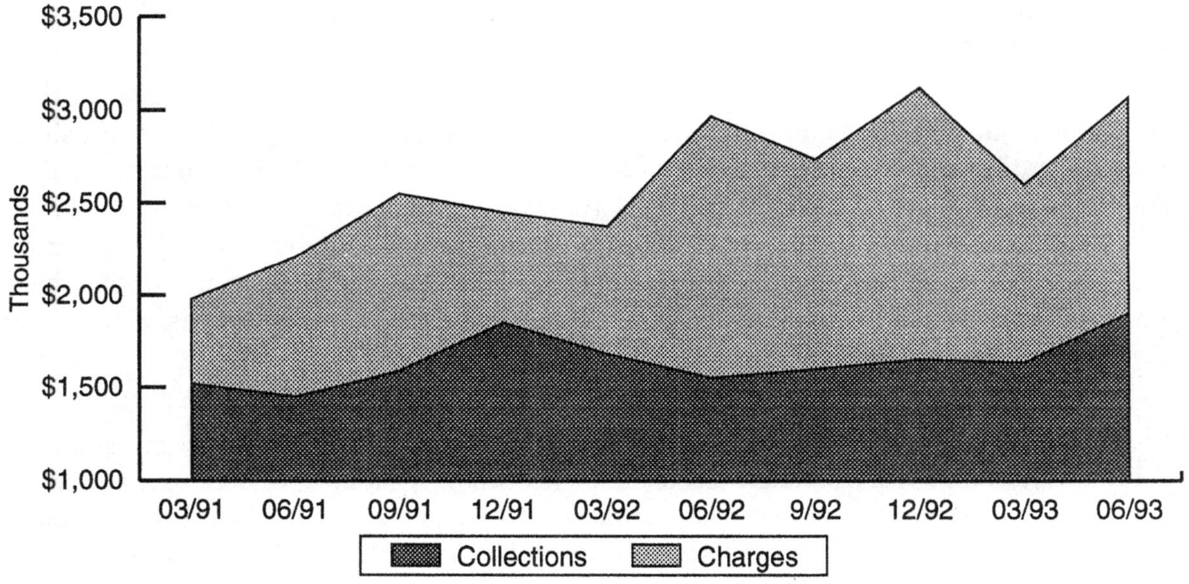

Figure 1–3 Charges to collections analysis.

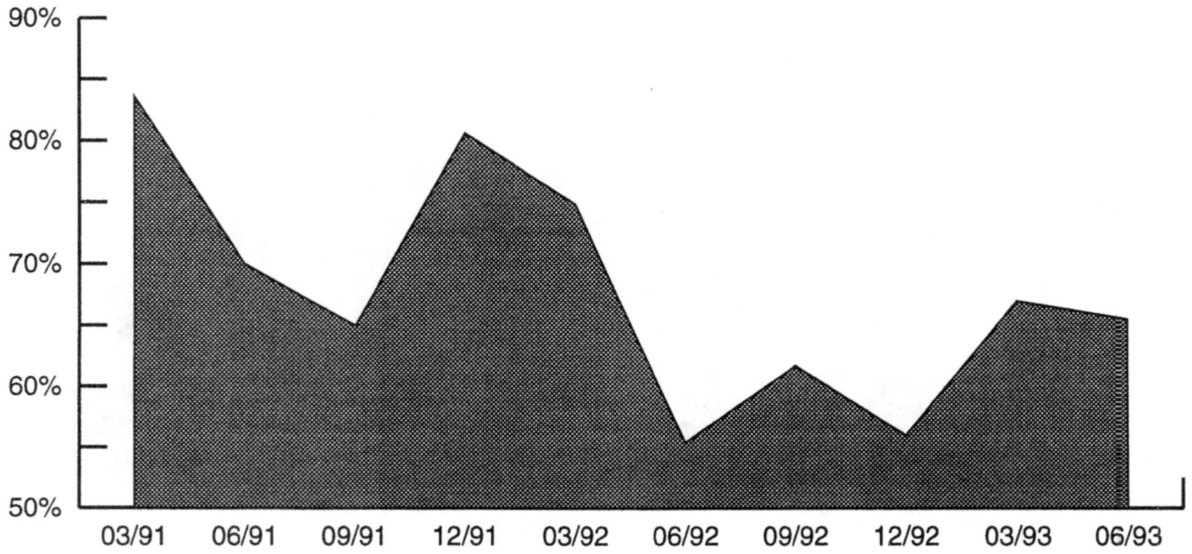

Figure 1–4 Collections as a percentage of charges.

A Quick Look at the Balance Sheet

Let's start with a quick look at the balance sheet. Refer to Exhibit 1–1. This particular balance sheet illustrates a basic point for medical practices: Their balance sheets should be straightforward. Assets should typically consist of cash, some furniture, fixtures, medical equipment, and perhaps an automobile. The liabilities on your balance sheet should be short-term obligations such as payroll taxes or pension contributions payable. The balance sheet should have long-term debts only if there is a corresponding asset associated with that debt. For instance, it would be proper to have bank loans payable on your balance sheet if the proceeds from the loans were used to purchase medical equipment. In your quick analysis, your key factors should be designed to isolate the three most common problems with medical practice balance sheets.

Problem 1: Practice money gets lost in the pipeline. Does your balance sheet show investments in stocks, bonds, or life insurance? It should not. Remember, your practice is a conduit. If your money gets invested before it gets to the other end of the pipeline, it will cause double taxation if your practice is incorporated. (This book assumes that your practice is incorporated. The last chapter will discuss why I believe that all medical practices should be professional corporations.)

Solution: Investments should be made by individuals, not by professional corporations.

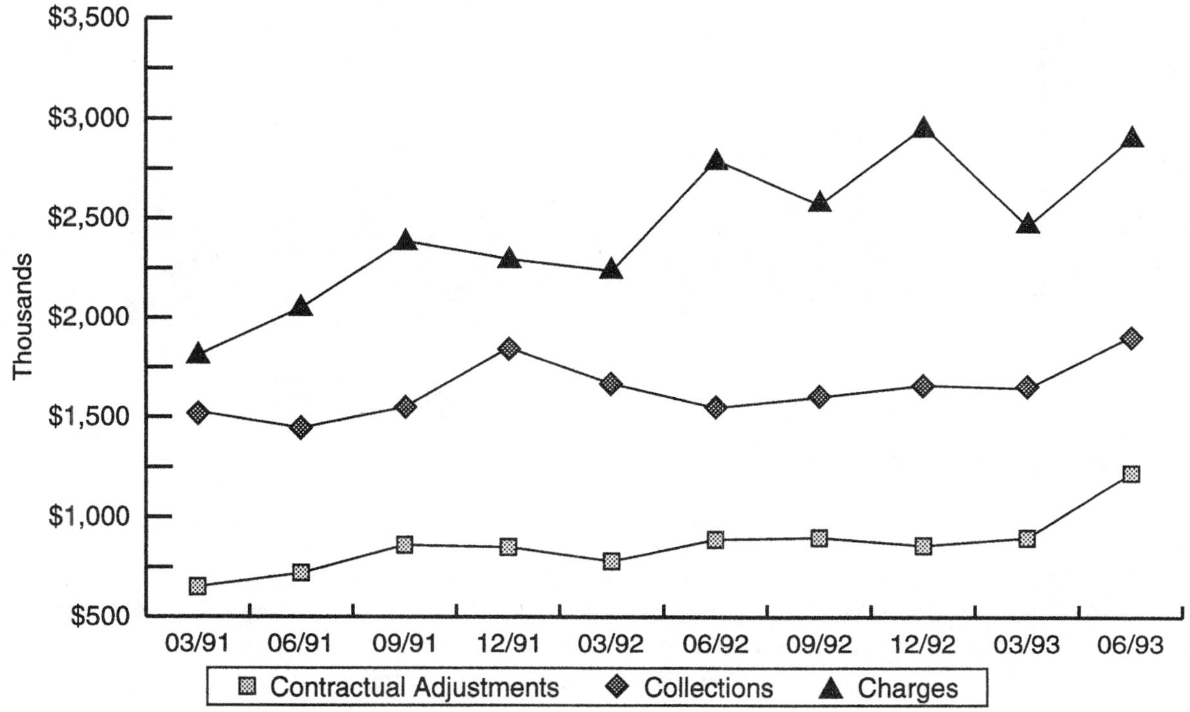

Figure 1–5 Charges, collections, and contractual adjustments analysis.

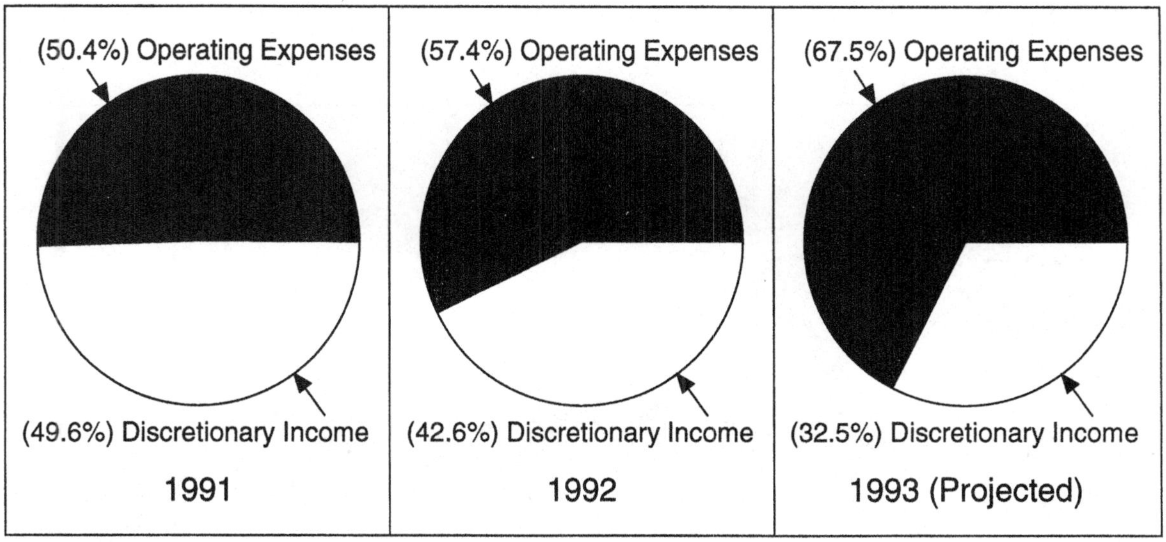

Figure 1–6 Analysis of operations, 1991–1993.

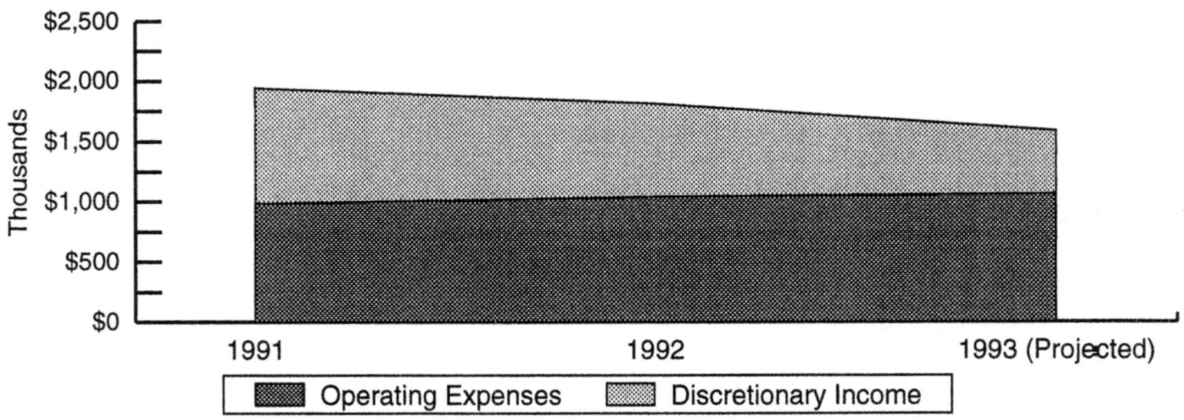

Figure 1–7 Analysis of operations.

Problem 2: Is there a loans-to-officers category on your balance sheet? If so, get rid of it. In recent years misguided advisors have often instructed physicians to borrow money from their professional corporations to avoid paying taxes. This is totally unacceptable advice. I have seen more than one physician stung by the onerous tax consequences of following it. Not only does this mistake cause double taxation (once at the corporate level and then later at the individual level), but quite often the Internal Revenue Service will take the position that the loan is in fact a nondeductible dividend paid to the physician. This is the worst tax consequence of all.

Solution: Do not borrow money from your professional corporation. If you already have, however, make sure that the loan is properly treated as compensation before the end of each fiscal year.

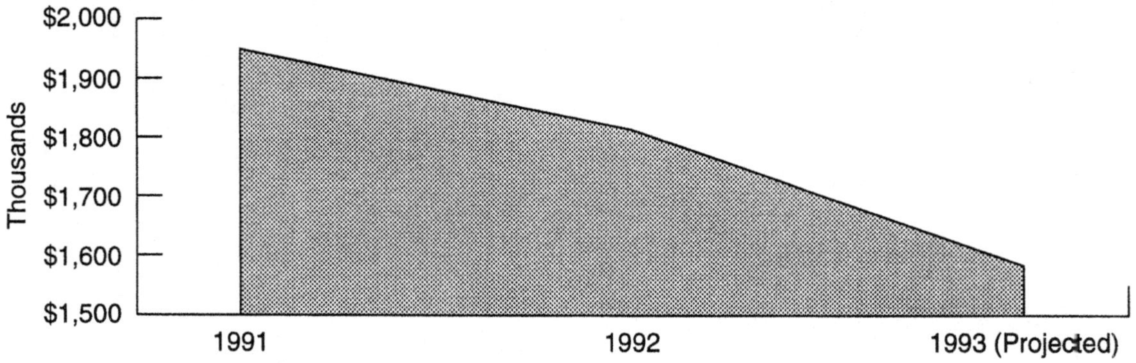

Figure 1–8 Analysis of net revenue received.

Problem 3: Look for loans that were not incurred to purchase assets but rather to pay ongoing operating expenses.

Solution: Never borrow money to pay operating expenses. Something is drastically wrong if a practice cannot pay its operating expenses from patient receipts. The problem needs to be identified and corrected. Trying to make problems go away by throwing borrowed cash at them is a short-term solution at best.

A Quick Look at the Income Statement

Now let's analyze some income statement key factors.

As you recall, the income statement should be divided into three sections: practice income, practice expenses, and physician compensation.

You and your accountant should identify your income statement key factors. These key factors must then be compared to standards so that you can develop expectations about how your practice should be operating. These practice expectations or goals are then continually monitored.

There is a wealth of readily available publications that will give you comparative information about these three sections of your income statement. These comparative data are available by specialty and by geographic region. Also, they are usually reported for single-specialty and multi-specialty groups.

A few good sources for obtaining comparative data are the following:

- *Medical Economics,* (800) 621-4431
- *Medical Economics for Surgeons,* (800) 621-4431
- *Cost Survey* and *Physicians' Compensation and Production Survey,* published by the Medical Group Management Association, 1355 South Boulevard, Suite 900, Denver, CO 80222, (303) 753-1111
- *Physicians Marketplace Statistics,* published by the American Medical Association, PO Box 109050, Chicago, IL 60610, (312) 464-5000
- Information compiled by the Society of Medical–Dental Consultants, (800) 826-2264
- Information published by the academy, association, or college that represents your specialty

By subscribing to a few of these references, you will be able easily to obtain the very important data necessary to determine how your practice compares with a variety of averages and parameters.

Section 1 of the Income Statement: Practice Income

Examine the practice income section of Exhibit 1–3 for the pediatric practice. As you can see, this practice collected approximately $269,000 in patient revenues per physician.

However, the national average for collections per pediatrician is about $304,000, which is significantly higher. There is a need to determine why this situation exists.

A key factor for the analysis of a medical practice's income statement is comparing collections per physician to national or regional averages for that specialty (your CPA or accountant should present comparative analytic data to you in concert with the preparation of your financial statements).

If collections per physician are significantly lower than average, it is generally attributable to one or more of the following problems:

- The practice's fee schedule is too low. This is a common problem that is addressed at length in Chapter 2.
- Accounts receivable are not being maintained properly, a very common and serious problem that is addressed in Chapter 3.
- The practice's patient mix needs to be improved.
- The practice may be experiencing employee theft.

Section 2 of the Income Statement: Practice Expenses

To establish key factors in this section, begin by comparing your practice's operating expenses, expressed as a percentage of your gross collections, with national or regional averages. This comparison will usually yield some interesting results.

First, compare the practice's total expenses with published averages. Is 60% of every dollar your practice collects consumed by operating expenses, when the regional average is 50%? If so, it is time to dig deeper to discover why.

Next, compare each major expense line item with established norms. This will help you develop a sense of what the practice's specific problems are.

Here are a few hints. The operating expense that most often gets out of control is nonphysician (staff) salaries. Always make it a key factor. If your staff salaries are several percentage points above average, then this may be an indication that further investigation is necessary. Are you paying your staff too much? Is your practice overstaffed? Is overtime being mismanaged?

Other expense categories that tend to become excessive are rent, office and medical supplies, and outside professional fees.

We will discuss in the next lesson what to do when expenses are out of control. For now, the important concept is being able to identify quickly how your practice's key factors compare with established benchmarks for your specialty.

Section 3 of the Income Statement: Physician Income

The key factor here is physician compensation compared with averages for your specialty. The *Physicians' Compensation and Production Survey* published by the Medical Group Management Association summarizes physician compensation. This excellent publication provides the mean, median, 10th, 25th, 75th, and 90th compensation percentiles by specialty.

Typically if physician compensation is below average, it is attributable, obviously, to the fact that practice income is too low and/or practice expenses are too high. You also need to ask one more question, however: Are all the practice's collections flowing through the pipeline? There are a couple of reasons why they may not be. The first reason is that cash gets stuck in the conduit. This problem was addressed when we discussed the balance sheet. Remember, the practice is a conduit: Get the cash through the pipeline and into physicians' pockets as soon as possible. Another reason why a physician's compensation may be below average is employee theft.

Not too long ago I was in Arizona on a consulting engagement. When I returned to my hotel, there was a frantic message from a new client in Florida that said he had a terrible problem. I called him back, and he began to tell me how his "most trusted" employee had systematically stolen more than $300,000 from his practice. There were many reasons why this theft went undetected; if this physician had known how his practice results compared with certain averages for plastic surgeons, however, he may have had some earlier indication that something was wrong and needed further investigation.

More than 50% of all medical practices will experience some form of employee theft in the form of money, drugs, or supplies. Equally unfortunate is the fact that the theft is usually executed by your most trusted employee. Be careful. Your accountant should help you set up and periodically test your system of internal accounting controls. Depending on the size of your practice, it may be necessary for you to get personally involved in some aspects of the practice's internal accounting control systems.

• • •

You have just learned one of the most important fundamentals of practice management. From now on, when you receive your timely and accurate financial statements, you will be able to analyze practice results quickly to determine your practice's strengths and weaknesses.

LESSON 1–5: FIND THE BAD NEWS, OR IT WILL SURELY FIND YOU

There is a big difference between having a vague feeling that something is wrong in your practice and having the numbers staring you in the face.

This lesson will teach you how to transform the problem areas uncovered in your comparative analysis into newly found dollars and cents. The lesson will focus on operating expense control. Chapters 2 and 3 will discuss correcting medical practice revenue problems.

A few years ago I was asked to perform a practice management review for a group of plastic surgeons. The group's problem on the surface was simple: The practice had significant gross revenue, but compared with salary averages for plastic surgeons, the physicians were earning comparatively little money. Their complaint was the one that I most often hear from physicians: "I'm working so hard, and yet I have nothing to show for it."

At first glance it appeared that this practice was doing everything right. The physicians had gorgeously appointed offices, their own surgical suites, and a highly trained and efficient staff. They were on the cutting edge of tasteful marketing. So, "How come we aren't making any money?"

One of the first steps I performed was to select key factors from their income statement and compare them with regional averages for plastic surgeons. As usually happens, problems came tumbling out of the woodwork. Several major expense categories were significantly above average. Rent, medical supply costs, advertising, anesthesiology charges, and staff salaries were all significantly above expectations.

I met with the physicians to discuss my initial findings. I could see that they understood what I was saying, but I also sensed they did not fully comprehend the significance of what was happening. It was then that I presented my findings in a format similar to Exhibit 1–6. This worked.

The form translated my concerns into dollars. The physicians realized that by controlling certain expenditures they could generate additional income of more than $500,000 for themselves without working any harder than they already were. How this was accomplished is discussed in the next lesson.

The lesson to be learned here is early diagnosis and treatment. As soon as you realize that something is wrong in your practice, begin the process of ferreting it out. Be specific. Using Exhibit 1–6, list all the key factors in your practice that are not meeting expectations, and translate those expense categories into dollars. Once problems are identified in black and white and the dollar significance is apparent, solving those problems becomes much easier.

Exhibit 1–6 Income Statement Analysis Summary

Practice Expenses Category	*Actual Key Factor (%)*	*Expected Key Factor (%)*	*Dollar Value Based on Collections*
Medical supplies	XX	X	$ 50,000
Advertising expense	XX	X	240,000
Staff salaries	XX	X	60,000
Anesthesiology expense	XX	X	100,000
Rent expense	XX	X	60,000
POTENTIAL PRACTICE DOLLARS TO BE RECOVERED:			$510,000

LESSON 1–6: SOMETIMES YOU NEED A SCALPEL AND SOMETIMES AN AXE

Knowing the difference is crucial.

I learned a lesson early in my career. When I first began consulting, I would write my report and send it to the physicians to read before I met with them. I thought this was a good idea because it gave them a few days to familiarize themselves with what we would discuss in detail when we met.

In fact, all I had done was poke a stick into a hornet's nest. The physicians, angered by the problems and loss of revenue outlined in the report, would pull out their broadswords and start swinging. By the time I got to the office, blood was everywhere. The survivors were giving me warning looks that it would not be a good idea for me to seek medical treatment in this office.

The lesson here is: Don't overreact. Problems develop over time. It will take time to solve them. Also remember that an overall goal of practice management is to build an efficient, motivated team to support the physician. Discernment is the crucial skill needed to reach this objective. Knowing when to encourage change and when to make radical changes is the key to transforming your practice successfully into an efficient, pleasant operation.

With that in mind, let's use the plastic surgery practice we discussed in the last lesson and continue the case study. As you recall, their expenses were out of line in the following areas: medical supplies, advertising, staff salaries, anesthesiology charges, and rents. As we worked to solve these problems, sometimes we used an axe, and sometimes we used a scalpel.

Medical Supplies

Pull out the scalpel. We discovered that this practice purchased all its pharmaceuticals and many of its medical supplies from the local pharmacy. No one in the practice was responsible for purchasing medical supplies. Whenever something was needed, an employee picked up the telephone and placed an order. The local pharmacist was nice and delivered promptly.

The first step was to assign the duty of medical supply purchasing to one knowledgeable nurse. All requests for supplies had to go through her. We explained to her the problems that the practice was experiencing in this area and gave her an incentive to solve these problems. As usually happens, she couldn't wait to take on the challenge. The nurse investigated wholesale medical supply houses and negotiated excellent prices for the practice. Additionally, she convinced a wholesaler to prepare sterile custom packs for the procedures most often performed by the practice. These packs gave the physicians exactly the supplies they needed for specific procedures and eliminated the waste of having to discard unused supplies. In area after area, this nurse found ways to cut medical supply costs because she was now a part of the process. Annual savings: $50,000.

Advertising Expense

The axe. This practice was truly on the cutting edge of medical marketing. Initially working with a moderate budget and a local advertising agent, the physicians were able to develop a marketing package that significantly increased their business. A $10,000 per month expenditure, however, was allowed to expand unchecked into a $35,000 per month expenditure. When I discussed this with the advertising agent, he became highly offended. Apparently, he felt that he was above questioning or anything so confining as a budget. His message to me was clear: He had made their practice, he was not replaceable, and he was now entitled to lifetime security. Bring out a very sharp axe.

It took very little persuasion on my part to convince the physicians that for $15,000 per month they could hire their own in-house, full-time marketing staff and still have adequate dollars remaining to continue to reach their market. Annual savings: $240,000.

Staff Salaries

The scalpel and the axe. There were several reasons why staff salaries were excessive. First, no one was really in charge of the staff. When this happens, staffs tend to expand geometrically over time. Also, overtime was being abused. The challenge here was to correct the problems at hand and to increase staff morale in the process. Staffing will be discussed in detail in Chapter 5. A brief summary of the solutions implemented follows.

First, the staff were organized and department heads created. Individuals who were not adequately performing their duties were terminated. This always creates a boost in the morale of your good employees because they are keenly aware of and disturbed by employees who refuse to carry their share of the work load.

Once the new staff were in place they were called together, and salary goals were discussed openly with them. Ideas were encouraged, and incentive systems based on overall practice operating results were put in place. Annual savings: $60,000.

Anesthesiology Expense

A scalpel, maybe even a laser. This plastic surgery facility contained its own ambulatory surgery unit that was staffed by outside anesthesiologists who were excellent and expensive. Our first step was to obtain the averages for what anesthesia services should cost for day surgery centers. We then discussed with the anesthesia group what anesthesia was currently costing and what it should be costing. After a few hours of negotiations, we were able to make the changes necessary to reduce the surgery facility's anesthesia costs to acceptable levels. Annual savings: $100,000.

Rent Expense

Neither the scalpel nor the axe worked here because an onerous lease had already been signed. What was needed was some creativity. The lease was for absolutely gorgeous space, but there was far too much of it. Because the number-one referring physician source for plastic surgeons is obstetricians and gynecologists, it was decided that we would recruit such a group to rent some of the practice's excess space.

Everybody won. The Ob-Gyns occupied prime space at very favorable terms. The plastic surgeons had a live-in source of referrals plus the added bonus of revenue generated by the Ob-Gyns using their surgical facility. Annual savings: at least $60,000.

Summary

This practice was able to improve its bottom line by more than $500,000 simply by identifying key factors, setting expectations, and then taking decisive positive action based on these expectations. At first there was some reluctance on the part of some of the physicians: "The pharmacist is nice," "Nurse Jones has been with us for a long time," "The anesthesiologists are great people," "We're just stuck with a bad lease," and so on. They decided to press on anyway, and now they all agree without question that they made the right decisions.

◆ **MEDICAL PRACTICE MANAGEMENT TRUTH 4** ◆

Never mold your practice around a problem. The best run practices are those that make the tough decisions.

LESSON 1–7: FINANCIAL STATEMENTS IN A NUTSHELL

Financial statements are your most important practice management tool and the foundation upon which management excellence is built. Here is the financial statement analysis process:

1. Customize
   - Develop financial statements that are tailor made for your practice.
2. Set preparation standards
   - Insist that financial statements be provided to you on time.
   - Insist that financial statements be accurate.
3. Identify key factors
   - Analyze your balance sheet:
     —Are asset categories proper?
     —Are liabilities and debts appropriate?
   - Analyze your income statement:
     —Are collections appropriate for your specialty?
     —How do practice expenses compare with averages for your specialty?
     —Is physician compensation appropriate for your specialty?
   - Identify practice weaknesses and the related dollar cost.
4. Develop expectations
   - Develop goals for identified practice weaknesses.
5. Solve the problem
   - Implement the solutions.
6. Monitor the process
   - Repeat this process every month or quarter depending on the size of your practice.

◆ Chapter 2 ◆

The Fee Setting Short Course

LESSON 2–1: PHYSICIANS CAN TALK ABOUT SEX EASIER THAN THEY CAN TALK ABOUT FEES

Two characteristics of physicians and their fees are sometimes baffling to me. The first is reluctance. Contrary to popular opinion, physicians hate to raise their fees. When I discuss fee increases with physicians, their faces turn ashen and their jaws begin to clench. This reaction always is followed by a litany of reasons explaining why it is not a good time to raise fees: "My patients will go to someone else," "The economy is bad," "The public already thinks we are greedy," "Colleagues will stop referring." None of which is true.

The truth is that most medical practices wait far too long to raise fees and then do so in a haphazard manner. One common method is to have an employee place a few phone calls to other practices to determine what they are charging. Another method is to apply a flat percentage increase to all procedures performed.

The result of these approaches to fee setting is that most medical practices' fee schedules are usually priced 10% to 20% below marketplace fee schedules. Eventually, these practices begin to feel the squeeze of inflation and are faced with making one large fee increase when several smaller ones over a period of time would have been much more palatable to everyone involved and more profitable for the physician.

The second baffling characteristic is physician passivity. Do you know of any other profession that so routinely has its fees involuntarily reduced and does nothing about it?

Imagine walking into your attorney's office and telling him or her, "You are bright, articulate, well educated, and highly trained. The work that you recently did for me was superb. I have looked over your fee schedule, however, and have decided to reimburse you at a rate of 65% of what you have charged me."

Have you ever considered going into Neiman Marcus and telling the salesperson, "I love this suit, but your price isn't reasonable or customary. Based on averages for all suits sold, this is the price I am going to pay."

Third party reimbursers are reducing physicians' fees more than ever before, and they will continue to do so because they are allowed to get away with it.

◆ MEDICAL PRACTICE MANAGEMENT TRUTH 5 ◆

A medical practice's fee setting strategy is an integral part of practice management.

In the previous chapter we discussed comparing collections for your practice with certain established averages. If your practice's collections are significantly below average, one or both of two factors may be responsible: Your fee schedule is inadequate, and/or your accounts receivable are not properly managed. We will discuss accounts receivable management in Chapter 3.

The purpose of this chapter is to establish an organized and easy-to-implement method of setting and monitoring medical fees. The lessons of this chapter will help you:

- Determine how your current fee schedule measures up to the market
- Set fees in a focused and organized manner
- Develop an annual fee review process

LESSON 2–2: A BLIND PERSON SHOULD ALWAYS KNOW WHERE HE OR SHE IS STANDING

Everyone has heard the old story about the enthusiastic, if not too bright, man who sold exquisite leather wallets at bargain prices too good to be true. One shopper asked, "Sir, how can you afford to sell wallets such as these so inexpensively?"

The man revealed his secret. "It's easy. I buy them direct from the factory for $10 and sell them to the public for $9."

"But how can you make any money buying wallets for $10 and selling them for $9?"

The man uttered just one word: "Volume."

An old story perhaps, but one worth repeating because I hear similar stories from physicians when I ask about pricing of certain procedures. Physicians use volume as an excuse for not raising fees. Physicians have told me that they purposely price certain procedures as loss leaders to attract new patients. It just does not work that way.

Numerous studies have shown that patient loyalty to physicians is not driven by price.

This lesson will discuss how to approach fee setting in a focused and organized manner. Your bookkeeper or office manager should complete the initial data gathering for setting fees. After the number crunching, you will be able to take the work product, review it, and use it to set fees in a relatively short period of time.

Relative Value Fee Setting

If you are like most practices, 20 to 30 CPT codes account for the majority of your charges. These are the procedures to which you want to pay particular attention when setting fees because changes here will have the most dramatic effect on your bottom line.

Exhibit 2–1 is a format for gathering basic fee schedule information. Take the top 20 to 30 procedures for your practice (those that account for 70% to 80% of dollar volume), and have your staff prepare a similar form.

Column 1: List the procedures to be analyzed.

Column 2: List each procedure's CPT code.

Column 3: List the annual volume for each procedure.

Column 4: List the present fee for each procedure.

Column 5: Compile the actual annual receipts for each procedure. These data should be readily available if your practice is computerized.

Column 6: Column 6 is the relative value units (RVUs) for each procedure. There are many source books for relative value units. I prefer *Relative Values for Physicians,* published by Systemetrics–McGraw-Hill, (800) 544-8168.

Exhibit 2–1 Format for Gathering Basic Fee Schedule Information

OB/GYNs MEDICAL CORP (APC)
RELATIVE VALUE FEE SCHEDULE

(1)	(2)	(3)	(4)	(5)	(6)	(7)	(8)	(9)	(10)	(11)	(12)
Procedure	CPT Code	Volume	Fee	Total $	RVU	100	125	150	175	Var @ 125	$ Effect
Routine obstetric care	59400	266	$1,675	$445,550	20	$2,000	$2,500	$3,000	$3,500	$825	$219,450
Routine care w/ c-section	59510	125	1,675	209,375	25	2,500	3,125	3,750	4,375	1,450	181,250
Postpartum tubal ligation	58605	43	750	25,325	8	750	938	1,125	1,313	188	8,063
Total abdominal hysterectomy	58150	39	1,800	70,650	17	1,700	2,125	2,550	2,975	325	12,675
Total vaginal hyst	58140	13	1,800	23,400	12	1,200	1,500	1,800	2,100	(300)	(3,900)
Exploratory laparotomy	49000	6	1,550	9,300	10	1,000	1,250	1,500	1,750	(300)	(1,800)
Laparoscopy diagnostic	58980	55	825	45,375	8	800	1,000	1,200	1,400	175	9,625
Lap tubal sterilization	58982	51	825	42,000	10	1,000	1,250	1,500	1,750	425	21,675
Salpingo oophorectomy	58720	8	1,550	12,400	11	1,140	1,425	1,710	1,995	(125)	(1,000)
Ectopic preg/exp lap	59120	2	1,550	3,100	14	1,400	1,750	2,100	2,450	200	400
D&C ob	59812	35	525	17,685	4	400	500	600	700	(25)	(875)
D&C gyn	58120	28	525	14,475	4	400	500	600	700	(25)	(700)
Conization of cervix	57520	49	675	32,625	5	500	625	750	875	(50)	(2,450)
Care of miscarriage	59820	9	525	4,725	5	450	563	675	788	38	338
Laser surgery office	57520	5	675	3,075	5	500	625	750	875	(50)	(250)
Salpingectomy	59120	4	1,550	6,200	14	1,400	1,750	2,100	2,450	200	800
Repair of enterocele	57268	2	1,700	3,400	10	1,000	1,250	1,500	1,750	(450)	(900)
Cystocele repair	57240	1	1,250	1,250	9	860	1,075	1,290	1,505	(175)	(175)
Vag hyst post & ant repair	58265	5	2,000	10,000	21	2,100	2,625	3,150	3,675	625	3,125
Marsupialization of cyst	56440	3	525	1,700	4	400	500	600	700	(25)	(75)
Annualized fee increase											$445,275

Columns 7 through 10: At the top of each column you see a number (such as 100, 125, and so on through 175). These numbers are conversion factors. There are several publications, such as *Medical Economics,* that provide a range of conversion factors based on specialty. I have selected the average conversion factor for obstetricians and gynecologists ($100) and various percentiles up to the 90th percentile ($175). The conversion factor is multiplied by the RVUs to provide a range of fees for each procedure.

Column 11: Based on the geographic location of this practice, we determined that the present fee schedule was well below the market and that a conversion factor of $125 was appropriate. Column 11 is the price difference between the current fee and the new fee at a conversion rate of $125. As you can see, some fees were increased and some were decreased.

Column 12 is the product of multiplying column 3 by column 11. The purpose of this calculation is to determine the total dollar effect on the practice once the new fee schedule is implemented. As you can see, this particular practice will experience an increase in charges of $445,275 without any patient growth. This is why proper fee setting is so important.

The relative value fee schedule takes the guesswork out of setting fees and is easy to adjust annually for inflation. It also provides you with a well-structured and organized method of reviewing and raising fees.

FEE SETTING TIPS

- Review and raise your fees annually by at least the rate of inflation.
- Try to keep your fees in the 75th to 90th percentiles for your area. The procedures that provide the most dollar volume should be charged out at the highest percentiles.
- A procedure in which you have particular expertise should always be valued at the highest possible conversion rate.

Don't be afraid to charge top dollar for your services. Remember that few of your fees will be paid in full. Between health maintenance organizations (HMOs), preferred provider organizations (PPOs), Medicare reimbursement rates, and reasonable and customary adjustments, you will be fortunate to collect 75% of your standard fee-for-service charges, so make sure your charges are as high as the marketplace will allow.

Fee Setting Summary Checklist

- Summarize the procedures that represent 70% to 80% of your practice's dollar volume.
- Assign CPT codes.
- Assign RVUs.
- Assign a range of conversion factors.
- Compare your current fees with an appropriate conversion factor for your location.
- Adjust your fees accordingly.
- Review and raise fees annually.

LESSON 2–3: RBRVS BY THE SAME PEOPLE WHO BROUGHT YOU THE IRS

Resource-based relative value scales (RBRVS): Doesn't that sound like a title only the government could create? But make no mistake, RBRVS are here, and one way or another they will have a serious impact on the way you practice medicine.

To explain RBRVS a little better, a short history lesson is in order. From 1975 to 1987 the government's cost per Medicare enrollee grew at a compounded annual rate of 15%. This growth rate was several times the rate at which the economy was growing as a whole. This infuriated our senators and congresspersons.

Ever vigilant, our elected representatives decided that they would not only slash Medicare reimbursements but would try to perform some social engineering as well. They created the new fee schedule to encourage more medical school students to become primary care providers rather than specialists and to attract more physicians to rural areas. They also intended to straighten out perceived inequities between the earnings of surgeons and primary care physicians. According to the Department of Health and Human Services, the purpose of RBRVS is to help address the long-standing imbalances between Medicare payments to urban and rural physicians and between primary care physicians and certain specialties, such as surgeons.

The purpose of this lesson is twofold. First, it will familiarize you with of the basics of RBRVS so that you can instruct your staff on how to calculate the effect of its implementation on your practice. If you have a high percentage of Medicare patients, it is important to know what your Medicare Fee Schedule (MFS) will be for the next several years. The second purpose is to hoist a red flag. If RBRVS succeed, they are a foreshadowing of economic pressures to come. Already insurance companies and managed care organizations are attempting to force similar reimbursement policies upon physicians.

The Basics of RBRVS

RBRVS establish relative values for more than 4000 medical services based on three factors:

1. *The physician work component RVU:* This component reflects the physician's expertise and expended efforts, with consideration being given to factors such as complexity, risk, and time associated with a procedure.
2. *The practice expense RVU:* This component reflects the practice overhead associated with a procedure.
3. *The malpractice cost component RVU:* This component reflects the malpractice cost associated with each medical service provided.

Each of these RVUs is adjusted by geographic factors that take into account the differing costs of conducting business in various parts of the country. These geographically adjusted RVUs are then multiplied by a dollar conversion factor published by the government. Let's look at the example in Exhibit 2–2.

The MFS is subject to certain phase-in rules, applied between now and 1996, depending on your current fee schedule. There also is a new limiting charge that replaces the maximum allowable actual charge for physicians who do not accept assignment. The limiting charge will be 20% above the Medicare fee schedule for 1992 and 15% for 1993 and beyond.

If your practice has a large number of Medicare patients, I recommend that you complete a spreadsheet summarizing the dollar effect that RBRVS will have on your medical practice as it is phased in (Exhibit 2–3). Be forewarned: You will be able to take some mitigating action.

By acting now, you can take steps to offset future loss of Medicare income and prepare your current fee schedule for upcoming battles with third party payers. What can you do? There are only three things that a medical practice can do to improve gross income:

- improve patient volume and mix
- provide a wider array of patient services
- raise fees for services performed.

Improving patient volume and mix will be discussed in Chapter 4. We've covered raising fees. How should you approach providing a wider array of services? First, keep up with new

---

Exhibit 2–2 Sample RVU Calculations

The components of the calculation:

A = CPT RVU
B = CPT Overhead RVU
C = CPT Malpractice RVU
D = Geographic Work Index
E = Geographic Overhead Index
F = Geographic Malpractice Index
G = Monetary Conversion Factor

The fee schedule formula:

$$(A \times D) + (B \times E) + (C \times F) \times G = \text{MFS}$$

The MFS for a total abdominal hysterectomy (CPT 58150) performed in New Orleans would be \$602 (compared with a standard fee of approximately \$1800), calculated as follows:

$$(9.57 \times 0.994) + (10.24 \times 1.003) + (2.22 \times 1.19) \times \$26.873 = \$602$$

Exhibit 2–3 MFS Effects

Procedure	CPT Code	Work RVU	Geograph Index	Practice RVU	Geograph Index	Malprac RVU	Geograph Index	Conversn Factor	MFS	Current Fee
Routine obstetric care	59400	13.800	0.994	7.900	1.003	1.490	1.185	26.873	$629	$1,675
Routine care w/ c-section	59510	17.140	0.994	12.140	1.003	2.580	1.185	26.873	867	1,675
Postpartum tubal ligation	58605	3.500	0.994	4.320	1.003	0.900	1.185	26.873	239	750
Total abdominal hysterectomy	58150	9.570	0.994	10.240	1.003	2.220	1.185	26.873	602	1,800
Total vaginal hyst	58140	8.080	0.994	8.060	1.003	1.640	1.185	26.873	485	1,800
Exploratory laparotomy	49000	9.540	0.994	7.090	1.003	1.470	1.185	26.873	493	1,550
Laparoscopy diagnostic	58980	3.900	0.994	4.910	1.003	1.060	1.185	26.873	270	825
Salpingo oophorectomy	58720	6.580	0.994	7.370	1.003	1.600	1.185	26.873	425	1,550
Ectopic preg/exp lap	59120	7.560	0.994	6.710	1.003	1.150	1.185	26.873	419	1,550
D&C ob	59812	3.290	0.994	3.100	1.003	0.670	1.185	26.873	193	525
D&C gyn	58120	2.000	0.994	2.890	1.003	0.610	1.185	26.873	151	525
Conization of cervix	57520	4.100	0.994	1.930	1.003	0.310	1.185	26.873	171	675
Care of miscarriage	59820	4.430	0.994	3.750	1.003	0.760	1.185	26.873	244	525
Laser surgery office	57520	4.100	0.994	1.930	1.003	0.310	1.185	26.873	171	675
Salpingectomy	59120	7.560	0.994	6.710	1.003	1.150	1.185	26.873	419	1,550
Repair of enterocele	57268	6.530	0.994	7.000	1.003	1.510	1.185	26.873	411	1,700
Cystocele repair	57240	5.720	0.994	5.620	1.003	1.120	1.185	26.873	340	1,250
Marsupialization of cyst	56440	2.970	0.994	2.680	1.003	0.540	1.185	26.873	169	525

technology; it will soon be more important to physicians than ever before. Lasers, scopes, and fiberoptics are making current procedures obsolete. Physicians must master new high-tech procedures as soon as they are accepted by the profession.

Furthermore, as unpalatable as it is to many physicians, medical practices of the future will sell pharmaceuticals, orthopedic devices, pediatric and maternity products, and other items. The purpose will be to raise revenue per patient, soon to be the new buzzword in medical practice management.

A Final Word

Write your elected representatives, and let them know how you feel about RBRVS before it's too late.

As an organized group, physicians could have political clout. The government still needs you more than you will need it. The threat of a nationwide strike would bring all third party payers back to the bargaining table in good faith. If medicine remains a confederacy of loosely aligned small practices, however, physicians will be picked off one by one over the next decade.

LESSON 2–4: MANAGING MANAGED CARE

Nothing illustrates more vividly what is happening in the practice of medicine today than the struggle taking place on the managed care battlefield.

As of now, most physicians are losing the war. If present trends continue, by the end of the century most physicians will be employees of large corporations, insurance companies, big provider groups, or hospitals. These large entities will have one common trait: They will be managed by businesspeople, whose primary focus will be making a profit.

The result of this new megamedicine will be that small independent practitioner groups will go the way of the house call. Practices that are not run in an efficient, businesslike manner will fail. Physicians who do not understand the business of medicine will earn significantly less than their peers.

◆ MEDICAL PRACTICE MANAGEMENT TRUTH 6 ◆

Physicians must understand and accept three realities to come to terms with managed care.

1. **Medicine is now big business.**
2. **The driving force behind managed care is profit.**
3. **Providers who learn to negotiate with managed care companies will fare best.**

What Is Managed Care?

Whether it is called an HMO, a PPO, a PHO, an individual practice association (IPA), or any other combination of letters, managed care is private enterprise's answer to a perceived problem.

For years the public has complained about the high cost of medical care and its limited availability to certain sectors of the population. Any time a problem involves billions of dollars, some bright entrepreneur will try to solve that problem and make a profit. This is how managed care was born.

Although managed care got off to a shaky start, it is now here to stay. Estimates are that by 1995, 50% of all patient care will be managed care.

In its simplest form, managed care is a contract. Businesspeople realized that they could make a profit if they could control patient use of medical services and the providers of those services. To obtain this control, they contracted with patients to provide specific medical services. This arrangement is nothing new. Now, businesspeople are contracting with physicians to provide services at predetermined prices and to provide services under certain controlled circumstances. Herein lies the new twist: control of both supply and demand. Clearly, managed care is just a business arrangement.

Tips for Living with Managed Care

Perform a practice analysis to determine which managed care organizations are best for your practice and which ones you are capable of serving. There are two main considerations here: market share and compensation.

Market share refers to how many patients the plan sends you. You should also consider the plan's ability to lock you into or out of a particular market. If you sign up with a plan, will you be the exclusive physician for your specialty in your area? Conversely, if you do not sign up with a plan will you lose a significant number of your existing patients? If you are a new physician trying to build a practice, you may consider signing up with almost every plan offered to you until your patient base is large enough for you to begin being more selective. In your early years it is better to see patients at 50 cents on the dollar than to have no patients at all. Additionally, these discounted patients will contribute to your fixed overhead.

Compensation is generally paid either as a capitated fee or as a percentage of your customary fee for service. Before signing up with a plan, you should complete the worksheet in Exhibit 2–4. This worksheet will provide you with an initial indication as to the appropriateness of the compensation being offered to you. If compensation appears reasonable, then you can proceed to analyzing the remainder of the contract as discussed in Part II.

Your attorney or CPA, along with a physician from your group, must learn how to negotiate contracts with managed care providers. All contracts are subject to negotiations, and certain sections should be closely scrutinized. Pertinent questions include the following:

- How and when will your group be compensated for services rendered? Ask for annual renegotiation of payment rates.
- What is the process for utilization review?
- What are the types of utilization pools, withholds, penalties, and/or bonuses in which you will participate? What is the plan's reputation for paying back withholds?
- What is the plan's philosophy regarding referrals to specialists? Obviously this is important if you are a specialist, but primary care physicians also need to know whether they will be pressured not to refer to specialists.
- How many lives does the plan cover, and which employers in your area are offering the plan?
- How many physicians in your specialty are already providers to the plan?
- What major industries does the plan represent?
- Is the plan financially sound? Check with your state's insurance commissioner to determine whether the plan has any serious complaints filed against it.
- Are other physicians currently in the plan happy with it?
- How do you terminate your relationship with the plan? You should ask for a 30- or 60-day without cause termination provision.

Exhibit 2–4 Compensation Worksheet for Managed Care Plans

1. Gross charges	__________
2. Less deductions:	
Fee discounts	__________
Withholdings	__________
Other deductions	__________
Total deductions	__________
3. Net charges	__________
4. Net collections	__________
5. Collection ratio	__________
6. Net charge ratio	__________

1. Gross charges are your usual and customary fee for services.
2. Deductions: Fee discounts are agreed upon reductions to your normal fee for services schedule. Withholdings are amounts withheld by the plan with a promise to pay back at a later time based on certain contractual criteria. Other discounts are items such as courtesy discounts to plan members.
3. Net charges are gross charges less total deductions.
4. Net collections are collections from all sources, including withhold payments.
5. The collection ratio is net collections divided by net charges. This percentage will give you an indication of the amount of your allowable charges for which you are being reimbursed. It should be between 90% and 100%.
6. The net charge ratio is net charges divided by gross charges. This percentage should be 70% to 75%.

- What is the range of services that you will be expected to provide and the hours that you must be available?
- Does the plan require you to be on any committees or make any other uncompensated demands upon your time?
- Are you required to indemnify the plan under any circumstances? Do not, unless the indemnification is mutual and the plan's liability insurer provides assurances that the indemnification is covered.
- What level of liability coverage is carried by the plan? Is the level of coverage that the plan requires you to carry reasonable?
- Does the plan require you to follow the same appointment and admitting procedures for its members as for your other patients? You may want to negotiate this option. Also, try to retain the option to close your practice to new plan members if you deem it necessary.

- Have you obtained and reviewed all documents that are referenced in the proposed contract? Have someone look closely at utilization review documents, quality assurance plans, and operating manuals to which you may be subject without realizing it.
- Is the plan physician friendly? Who determines medical necessity and defines an emergency condition? Is there a phone number for provider questions? Will someone from the plan spend some time providing initial training for your staff? Is it easy to verify patient eligibility?

Learn how to negotiate the best deal for your practice. Realize that there is strength in numbers. It has been my experience that the bigger the physician group, the better the terms it can negotiate with managed care organizations.

Future Shock

The future is bringing large organizations into the business of medicine. These organizations fall into two categories, and physicians will be working for one or the other.

The first type is the big corporation. In a continuing effort to cut costs, large corporations will directly employ physicians. How? Hospitals, insurance companies, and other organizations seek to capture an ever increasing share of the marketplace. The best way to do this will be to control a wide array of services. It will not be unusual for large corporations to own health insurance companies, HMOs, PPOs, hospitals, and home health care facilities. They also will hire the physicians needed to staff them.

The second type of organization will be the large multispecialty clinics that will evolve from physicians' efforts to compete with big business. If physicians retain any autonomy, this is the direction from which it will come.

Physicians who band together to form large multispecialty clinics offering a wide array of services (laboratory testing, radiology, and ambulatory surgical facilities) may be able to muster enough clout to control their professional lives. The key to these clinics' success will be efficiency. They must be administered as businesses as well as fine medical facilities.

Physicians who will thrive in this environment to come will be those who see the new horizons now and begin to position themselves and their practices for doing business in the 21st century.

LESSON 2–5: FEE SETTING IN A NUTSHELL

The medical economic frontier is scary. The federal government has already begun its attack on the medical profession. Its demands include not only fee control but control of which specialty you select and where you practice. Big business is more pragmatic, opting instead to control the marketplace and take its profits from patient and physician control. Meanwhile, the small practice still staggers from the onslaught of it all.

Now is the time to take action by developing short- and long-term strategies.

Short-Term Strategies

Review your practice's current fee schedule. To maximize changes, physicians must begin to analyze fees in a logical and organized manner. Remember that inflation never takes a rest. Fees must be adjusted annually by at least the rate of inflation.

Consider the effect of RBRVS on your practice, and develop a plan now to increase revenue per patient.

Long-Term Strategies

Learn everything you can about managed care, including how to negotiate the best contracts for your practice. Develop a five-year plan for your practice as well as strategic alliances with other physicians. Finally, consider merging your group with others to develop multispecialty clinics or IPAs that can compete in the marketplace of tomorrow.

◆ Chapter 3 ◆

The Accounts Receivable Short Course

LESSON 3–1: UNTIL IT'S CASH, IT'S ONLY PAPER

The newest catch phrase in medical practice management appears to be *cash flow*. Articles tell you how to enhance it. Consultants guarantee that they can improve it. To me, it's a new spin on the same old question, "I'm working so hard, where is all my money?" This question is often answered in two words: accounts receivable.

Sooner or later, every medical practice will be penalized by inefficient accounts receivable management. There are three reasons for this phenomenon:

1. Physicians are healers and "just want to practice medicine."
2. Physicians perceive collecting money as distasteful and unprofessional.
3. Physicians don't understand their role in the accounts receivable process.

These are all understandable reasons for physicians to avoid dealing with accounts receivable. Nevertheless, they must be weighed against this fact:

◆ MEDICAL PRACTICE MANAGEMENT TRUTH 7 ◆

No one will ever be as concerned about your money as you.

No one—your patients, your best employees, your attorney, or your CPA—can ever care as much about your receivables as you should. You must be involved continually in the accounts receivable process if your practice is to operate smoothly.

This chapter covers the physician's role in the accounts receivable process. It outlines the basics of accounts receivable and teaches you how to monitor its key factors:

- patient charges and payments
- contractual adjustments
- bad debt write-offs
- collection policies
- the importance of the Big Picture.

Monitoring accounts receivable is not time consuming. By hiring good employees and by properly delegating certain accounts receivable functions, the physician will be able to monitor his or her accounts receivable in about an hour each month. This hour may very well prove to be the most financially rewarding hour you spend in your practice.

LESSON 3–2: YOU CAN PAY ME NOW OR PAY ME LATER, MAYBE

Unless you are in a specialty fortunate enough to collect most of its fees at the time service is performed, your practice will constantly struggle with accounts receivable management.

The concept of accounts receivable seems simple. The physician provides the patient with medical services. For one of many reasons, the physician is to be paid at a later date. So far this is basic, uncomplicated commerce. At this point the chase begins.

Your Staff's Role in the Accounts Receivable Process

I will not go into great detail about your staff's role in the accounts receivable process. There are many excellent books and courses on this subject. Briefly, it is your staff's responsibility to do the following:

- Collect the maximum amount of charges at the time of service. This includes all copayments, deductibles, and charges for uninsured procedures.
- Verify insurance coverage before procedures are performed.
- Verify that all procedures have been properly coded by the physician on claims forms.
- Ensure that all claims forms are filed with third party payers within five days of the time of service.
- Properly record all charges, collections, contractual adjustments, and bad debt write-offs.
- Age and balance accounts receivable at the end of each month.
- Properly follow up on past due accounts and enforce all collection procedures.
- Prepare the appropriate accounts receivable analysis reports.

These responsibilities may sound straightforward, but don't let the simplicity fool you. It takes training and hard work for your staff to accomplish them efficiently. Be prepared to send your staff to several courses on CPT coding, insurance claims forms preparation and follow up, accounts receivable management, and billing and collection procedures. Your practice will more than recoup the cost of this training, however.

Additionally, your accountant must establish some basic internal accounting controls to verify the accuracy of data prepared by the staff and to minimize opportunities for employee misappropriation.

I cannot emphasize too strongly how important it is to train your staff properly and to establish proper internal accounting controls for accounts receivable. Poorly maintained accounts receivable systems lose money and provide significant opportunities for theft. Efficient accounts receivable systems provide excellent cash flow and patient satisfaction.

The Computer's Role in the Accounts Receivable Process

Accounts receivable management is one of the areas in a medical practice that will most lend itself to computerization. Computerization of accounts receivable will dramatically improve efficiency by:

- reducing human errors
- accelerating the filing of insurance claims forms
- accelerating the monthly closing of accounts receivable
- allowing the practice to age its accounts receivable easily
- allowing the staff to follow up easily on past due accounts
- allowing the practice to gather statistical data easily regarding patient referral sources
- allowing the practice to gather statistical data easily on which procedures are performed most often and which procedures generate the most dollar volume
- providing the practice with excellent demographic data on its patient base.

The Physician's Role in the Accounts Receivable Process

Each month, the physician must review two important reports and take appropriate action: the accounts receivable summary report, and the aged accounts receivable report.

Your staff should prepare these reports, but the physician must review them. Larger practices should select one physician for this important responsibility. The physician uses these reports to monitor practice performance, quickly spot billing and collection problems, and set practice goals to improve cash flow.

The Accounts Receivable Summary Report

Exhibit 3–1 is an example of the accounts receivable summary report. It summarizes all the activity in accounts receivable during the month. Details are not as important here as trends and common sense analysis. As you can see, this report provides you with the following practice information:

Beginning accounts receivable balance for the month
  (plus) Charges for the month
  (less) Collections for the month
(less) Contractual adjustments for the month
(less) Bad debt write-offs and professional courtesies
(equals) Ending accounts receivable balance for the month

Exhibit 3–1 Accounts Receivable Summary Report

Year	Charges	Receipts	1992–1993 Contractual Adjustments	Bad Debt Adj	Other Adj	Ending Accounts Receivable Balance	Gross Moving Average*		Net Moving Average†	
							12 mo	3 mo	12 mo	3 mo
1992										
Jan	103,443	(47,177)	(15,068)	(135)	1,476	249,323				
Feb	68,875	(57,407)	(37,923)	(470)	(101)	222,296				
Mar	71,104	(49,778)	(29,577)	(638)	627	214,034				
Apr	85,661	(38,932)	(19,800)	(4,065)	875	237,772				
May	70,156	(52,433)	(40,800)	(877)	(52)	213,764				
June	98,901	(63,644)	(37,873)	(3,961)	(339)	206,847				
July	69,015	(51,965)	(25,112)	(2,797)	(110)	195,876				
Aug	87,004	(55,266)	(38,287)	(7,186)	1,551	183,692				
Sept	84,828	(57,225)	(17,166)	(3,919)	1,128	191,337				
Oct	36,919	(52,891)	(26,816)	(8,607)	2,921	142,863				
Nov	69,197	(59,362)	(20,943)	(1,217)	2,329	132,868				
Dec	74,927	(39,049)	(10,860)	(236)	1,110	158,761	67.9%	83.6%	102.7%	116.0%
1993										
Jan	47,493	(48,263)	(14,346)	(2,271)	252	141,121	72.5%	76.5%	109.4%	101.0%
Feb	46,209	(37,284)	(11,577)	(2,069)	38	136,437	72.0%	73.8%	106.8%	95.7%
Mar	76,726	(49,647)	(15,302)	(2,838)	(762)	144,614	71.5%	79.3%	88.5%	103.5%
Apr										
May										

*Gross moving average = receipts divided by charges.

†Net moving average = receipts plus contractual adjustments divided by charges.

The physician's role is to check this report for propriety. Quite frankly, you are testing this information to determine whether it passes the common sense test. Ask yourself, "Does any part of this report not make common sense?"

For instance, make sure that the beginning of the month accounts receivable balance is the same number as the previous month's ending balance.

Review patient charges for the month, and ask yourself whether this total seems too high or too low based on how busy the practice was that month. If you have questions, ask for the summary of charges by day that make up total patient charges. Look it over. Does it seem reasonable?

Review patient collections for the month. Do they seem appropriate? Do patient collections on the accounts receivable summary report equal the total cash deposited into the bank that month? If not, find out why.

Review contractual adjustments. Every adjustment should be approved by a physician before it is written off. Ask to review each individual adjustment that makes up the monthly total. Review how much was written off, why it was written off, and who approved it.

Review bad debt write-offs in the same manner as contractual adjustments. Check the amounts written off, and check for the appropriate physician approval for doing so.

If any of the above categories do not pass the common sense test, you or someone outside your practice should investigate until you are satisfied that all aspects of accounts receivable are being handled properly.

It is also very important to keep collection trend information about your practice. This enables you quickly to spot a downward trend and determine its cause.

A downward trend in the gross or net ratios between charges and collections may indicate the following:

- Third party reimbursements, such as Medicare, are being cut.
- Your accounts receivable staff are not properly following up on past due accounts.
- There may be employee theft.
- Claims forms are not being properly prepared and submitted.

On the other hand, if you have had problems in the past, an uptrend in your gross collection ratio may indicate that the practice is on the road to correcting past problems.

Each month, take a few minutes to review your practice's collection ratio trend.

You will be richly rewarded with a practice that maximizes cash flow and minimizes opportunities for theft. You will be able to detect problems before they become disasters.

The Aged Accounts Receivable Report

The aged accounts receivable report is a list of every patient who owes the practice money. Its details typically include how much money is due and how long the balance has been owed. Exhibits 3–2 to 3–4 are examples of aged accounts receivable reports.

Exhibit 3–2 Aged Accounts Receivable Report: Summary Aging by Physician

SUMMARY AGING REPORT BY PHYSICIAN BASED ON DATE TREATED
Sydney Carrington & Associates P.A.
Sydney Carrington, MD (3)
All Physicians
Aging Category: 1–5/DOL Pay <= 04/12/93

Acct #	Name	Phone No.	DOL Pay	Current	31–60	61–90	91–120	120+	Total Balance
10	Carlson, Steven W	(916) 988-3293	04/11/90	92.95		202.20	5.80	107.70	408.65
14	Evans, Deborah A	(916) 678-5674	02/09/90	48.00		113.00			161.00
30	League, Claire E	(916) 907-4532	01/31/90			35.00		38.80	73.80
34	Dudley, Wayne R	(916) 789-6654	02/09/90					170.00	170.00
40	Green, Gordon R	(916) 334-5628	12/03/89	30.50		267.00		151.50	449.00
45	Williamson, Grant E	(916) 543-3344	01/04/90			48.00			48.00
90	Devoe, Lucia R	(916) 694-9528	04/11/90	89.00					89.00
110	Evans, Patricia G	(916) 544-8275	02/09/90			37.80	14.04		51.84
120	Williams, Terry L	(916) 875-3256		150.00	28.00				178.00
	REPORT TOTALS			410.45	28.00	703.00	19.84	468.00	1629.29
	PERCENT OF TOTAL AGED			25.2%	1.7%	43.1%	1.2%	28.7%	

Reprinted with permission of Systems Plus Inc® from their *The Medical Manager®* software.

This report requires a bit more of the physician's time. Depending on the specialty, physicians can expect to be paid for services rendered 60 to 90 days after filing a claim. Once an account is 120 days old, the chances of ever being paid drop dramatically.

To minimize accounts receivable losses, it is the physician's responsibility to ensure that the following procedures are performed:

- The accounts receivable clerk must prepare the aged accounts receivable report within 10 working days after the end of each month.
- The accounts receivable clerk must be assigned, in writing, the task of following up on past due accounts. Send the clerk to at least one seminar on credit and collection procedures for medical practices.
- Without fail, the physician must meet with the accounts receivable clerk every month and discuss the status of every account over 90 days old.
- Take action! Follow up with insurance companies, call patients to arrange payment terms, and decide what to do with patients who refuse to pay. Generally, if a patient truly

Exhibit 3–3 Aged Accounts Receivable Report: Summary Aging—Insurance Due Only

SUMMARY AGING REPORT BY INS CO BASED ON DATE INSURANCE BILLED
Sydney Carrington & Associates P.A.
Sydney Carrington, MD (3)
All Ins Cos
Aging Category: 1–5/DOL Pay <= 04/12/93

Co #	Name	Phone No.	Current	31–60	61–90	91–120	120+	Total Balance
1	Blue Cross/Blue Shield	(800) 345-7689			290.00			290.00
2	Beneficial Industrial Co	(800) 654-2323			35.00			35.00
3	Medicare Plus	(800) 675-4354			33.60	10.80	93.60	138.00
4	Employees Trust Insurance	(312) 456-7865			129.60			129.60
5	Aetna Life & Casualty	(800) 908-7654			107.64		126.00	233.64
6	Nationwide Health Insur	(213) 456-7654			5.80	12.80		18.60
7	Medicare	(800) 879-6789			750.00	90.00		840.00
8	Medi-Cal Insurance	(415) 987-0987	95.00		733.00		76.50	904.50
9	Fringe Benefit Center	(800) 678-0943	48.00					48.00
10	Champus	(800) 552-6612	3103.00	289.00	131.00		330.00	3,853.00
	REPORT TOTALS		3246.00	289.00	2215.64	113.60	626.10	6,490.34
	PERCENT OF TOTAL AGED		50.0%	4.5%	34.1%	1.8%	9.6%	

**** Report Does Not Include UNBILLED Insurance Items ****

Reprinted with permission of Systems Plus Inc® from their *The Medical Manager®* software.

Exhibit 3–4 Aged Accounts Receivable Report: Practice Aging Analysis

SYSTEM AGING ANALYSIS BY PHYSICIAN
Sydney Carrington & Associates P.A.
Summary for Practice

Type	Current	31–60	61–90	91–120	120+
Patient	90.95	28.00	70.90	132.50	415.50
%	12.3%	3.8%	9.6%	18.0%	56.3%
Insurance	2,787.20	2,672.00	2,855.64	113.60	626.10
%	30.8%	29.5%	31.5%	1.3%	6.9%
Totals	2,878.15	2,700.00	2,926.54	246.10	1041.60
%	29.4%	27.6%	29.9%	2.5%	10.6%

Total Patient Receivables	—	737.85	7.5%	(Date-Patient-Responsible)
Total Insurance Receivables	—	9,054.54	92.5%	(Date-Company-Billed)
Total Open Items	—	9,792.39	100.0%	(Summation-of-Above)
Unapplied Credits	—	30.00		
Total Accounts Receivable	—	9,762.39		

Reprinted with permission of Systems Plus Inc® from their *The Medical Manager®* software.

cannot pay you should write off the account balance and consider it pro bono work. What if a patient can pay but refuses? Accounts with small balances should be turned over to a reputable collection agency. Talk to an attorney about accounts with large balances.

The key to good accounts receivable management is having a well-trained staff who know that the physician is regularly involved in and is keenly interested in the results of their work.

LESSON 3–3: ACCOUNTS RECEIVABLE IN A NUTSHELL

The billing and collection process, or accounts receivable, as it is usually called, is the lifeblood of your practice. Yet it is often approached in a haphazard manner. Worse, it is totally ignored until major cash-flow problems arise.

I am sympathetic to physicians who "just want to practice medicine," but you still must do your part. Take an hour each month to perform the physicians' accounts receivable ten, no matter what. If you do these ten things, I can virtually assure you that you will never have an accounts receivable problem.

1. Pay whatever it takes to hire the best insurance and accounts receivable clerks. Generally, paying 10% above the market rate for employees will allow you to attract and keep the best and brightest employees.
2. Pay for them to attend classes on CPT coding, insurance claims forms processing and filing, billing and collection procedures, and accounts receivable management.
3. Set practice collection goals each month, and give your staff incentives to attain them. There are any number of incentives that can be put in place in your practice. For instance, your office manager may receive an incentive bonus based on overall practice results. Part of that bonus may be based on quarterly collections. Another example would be an incentive bonus for your accounts receivable department based on the staff's ability to equal or exceed expected collection ratios for your specialty compared with regional or national averages. Be careful: Once you have an incentive plan in place, it is sometimes hard to terminate it without causing morale problems, so be sure your plan is well thought out.
4. Manage the practice's insurance claims filing and accounts receivable on a computer.
5. Insist that accounts receivable be closed and balanced and that all the reports discussed in this chapter be prepared no later than ten working days after the end of each month.
6. Poke around. Without being obvious about it, take a look at patient charges one day each week. On another day, look at patient collections and the bank deposit slip. On another, review any write-offs or professional courtesy adjustments.
7. Closely review the accounts receivable summary report. Watch for trends, and check out any items that do not make sense.
8. Closely review the detailed aged accounts receivable report, and take action on past due accounts.
9. Closely review gross and net collections moving averages. Any unhealthy trends must be investigated.
10. Be involved in accounts receivable. It is your money. The concern that you exhibit will be mirrored by your staff.

◆ Chapter 4 ◆

The Short Course on Competition

LESSON 4–1: WHAT YOU AND A MERCEDES BENZ HAVE IN COMMON

For years, you seldom saw a Mercedes Benz ad. Then BMW introduced an intense advertising campaign aimed directly at the Mercedes market share. The Japanese decided that they, too, wanted a piece of the luxury car market. They introduced Lexus and Infiniti with comprehensive marketing strategies.

Within two years, Lexus replaced Mercedes at the top of customer satisfaction and quality surveys. Several pretenders to the luxury car market throne disappeared. Competition became fierce. Suddenly, there were too many luxury car manufacturers chasing too few buyers.

Now, you see plenty of Mercedes Benz advertising. There are tasteful spots on television, beautiful print ads, and special mailers directed to target markets. There is a lesson here for physicians.

For many years, physicians could rely on word of mouth and reputation to build excellent practices. Those days are drawing to an end as more and more predators move into your marketplace. In many communities today, there are too many physicians and too few patients.

◆ MEDICAL PRACTICE MANAGEMENT TRUTH 8 ◆

Competition is going to force marketing onto the practice of medicine.

Practices that flourish in the future will be those that have mastered the art of winning the hearts and minds of their patients.

Neil Baum, MD, full-time urologist, noted speaker, and author of *Marketing Your Clinical Practice* [(800) 638-8437], continually stresses the point that the successful private practices of the future will be those that place a premium on making the patient feel special.

What will be the key to competing? Marketing!

Before we go further, let me point out that you already market. Every time you walk into an examination room, you are marketing. Every time someone answers the telephone at your office, you are marketing. Every time someone walks into your waiting room, every time a patient's relatives want to talk to you, each and every time you or your staff make contact with a fellow human being, it is marketing.

The question is: How well are you managing your marketing? Marketing is a never ending process that involves every member of your staff. Each situation above is a moment of truth. How you manage these critical moments to make a good impression on your patients will ultimately determine much of your success.

This chapter is dedicated to convincing you, the practicing physician, of the importance of developing a marketing plan. This plan needs to consist of two major elements: internal and external marketing.

Internal marketing deals with the variety of actions that you and your staff use to present a polished, caring, and efficient image to current patients and referring physicians. External marketing includes those actions that you and your staff use to attract new patients and referral sources by getting the word out that yours is a polished, caring, and efficient practice.

There are many reasons to develop a marketing plan:

- Most important, it will make your practice a winning contender in a fiercely competitive marketplace.
- A marketing plan will force you to write specific goals for future growth, target markets, image, efficiency, and specialized services.
- A marketing plan will help you discover your strengths and weaknesses as well as perceptions about your practice of which you may be unaware.
- A marketing plan will define ways to enhance the good will of current patients and to attract new patients.
- Finally, a marketing plan will help you develop and maintain a dependable referral base.

Does a marketing plan work? Absolutely.

Two years ago I was asked to participate in the development and implementation of a marketing plan for a large obstetrics and gynecology group. This group of physicians believed that the local economy was sluggish and that it would not soon improve. They also saw that medicine was changing and that, if they were to prevent their patients from slipping away, they must become much more aggressive in the marketplace. The practice hired a medical marketing firm. The first step was gathering information. The firm interviewed physicians and staff about their needs and desires. They surveyed patients and noted their impressions about the practice. They reviewed demographics of the surrounding area to determine the potential patient mix.

The next step was developing internal and external marketing plans with which the physicians could be comfortable. The firm proposed several ideas, some as simple as adopting a corporate logo and coordinating stationery and brochures to create a practice identity. Others, such as staff training programs, tasteful advertising, and implementation of a new patient-oriented mentality, were more involved. Each physician in the group committed to good faith implementation of a plan drawn from these ideas.

The result? Although the economy continued to languish, the practice experienced a renaissance. New physicians had to be recruited to handle growth, patients were happier with the treatment provided by the "new" practice, employees experienced new found pride in their organization, and the physician/owners experienced a 66% increase in salary. Not bad.

Sometimes good marketing results from a single idea. A urologist concerned about undetected prostate cancers wrote a letter explaining the advantages of early detection by means of a simple blood test. He stuffed it into his monthly statements.

As a result, 75 patients came in for the test including eight new patients to whom the information had been passed along. The urologist detected three cancers and performed two radical prostatectomies. This simple mailing to 250 patients produced $20,000 in revenue for the practice.

Does marketing work? You bet, and it can save lives as well!

LESSON 4–2: YOU ALREADY HAVE THE BEST MARKETING PEOPLE IN THE WORLD WORKING FOR YOU

Your staff.

Here are some interesting facts. Surveys show that the number one reason patients change physicians is to obtain better service. One dissatisfied patient will tell up to 20 potential patients about an unpleasant experience at your practice. A satisfied patient will only tell 3 people about the pleasant experience. Bad news spreads quickly, but getting the good news out is much more difficult.

By far, the most effective and least costly method of marketing is internal marketing. Every day, you and your staff have several critical contact points. Contact points are those times when you have the opportunity to relay a positive message to patients, physicians, nurses, and anyone else who will form an opinion about you and your practice. Internal marketing includes everything you can do to ensure that these opinions are positive. It encompasses the entire effort put forth by your team to guarantee an image of excellence, in substance and form.

The elements of your internal marketing plan can be varied. They can be as simple as making sure that your telephone is always answered with a compassionate voice and as complex as hiring image consultants to put together a corporate identity package. Simple or complex, your internal marketing plan should be creative. In the long run, no one knows your patients as well as you and your staff. Put your heads together to determine what your patients need and how you can deliver it.

Three Steps to Internal Marketing

Step 1: Information Gathering

Some ideas about how to begin this process are as follows:

- Analyze your current patient base in terms of age, gender, and income. Compare the results with the same information for your community. Any segment of the community that your practice is not reaching could be a target group.
- Conduct a public opinion survey to determine how many people in your area are familiar with your practice and what impressions they have of it.
- Conduct patient surveys to find out how the practice is performing. Are patients satisfied with your services? Would they refer a friend to this practice? Were they treated properly by you and your staff?
- Survey your staff, and have regular meetings with them. They can tell you a great deal, such as what your patients really think and how the practice can be improved. You also

should be interested in how your staff feels that you treat them. As a general rule, how well you treat your staff is reflected in how well they treat your patients and referral sources.
- Use "mystery patients" for feedback about how your practice performs. Have a friend call your practice or see you as a patient and relay their experience to you.

Step 2: Deciphering Data

Use the results of your analysis to identify target markets and to set specific marketing goals. Quantify your expectations.

Step 3: Develop the Internal Marketing Plan

All physicians in your group must be comfortable in committing themselves to all parts of the final plan. Examples of what some practices have included in the marketing plan are as follows:

- Develop patient information brochures on a variety of pertinent topics.
- Develop a practice brochure to introduce the physicians and the practice to patients.
- Develop a patient relations protocol. Set standards for telephone communications, patient scheduling, and solving patient problems. Little details here make a big difference in how patients perceive your practice. Every employee should give the impression that "we care" about the experience each patient has at "our" practice.
- Develop a protocol or a list of standards for how physicians in your practice deal with patients. Again, little things will set your practice apart: Return calls promptly, be on time, don't talk down to patients, don't talk to patients with your hand on the doorknob. Develop a patient-centered protocol for all types of patient communications.
- Develop a practice identity package. Coordinate all your stationery, handouts, booklets, and even uniforms for your staff. Make your office decor pleasant, inviting, and patient friendly.
- Develop a practice logo and, if appropriate, a slogan.
- Have a physician or nurse call patients at critical times, such as after an operation or after starting a new treatment. A simple call that tells the patient after the service has been rendered that someone cares works wonders.
- Develop a list of drug stores where your patients can purchase prescriptions least expensively.
- Have patient focus groups. A couple of times a year, invite a representative number of patients to your office for lunch. Have your office manager ask them for opinions and recommendations for your practice.

- Conduct exit interviews of patients who leave your practice. This could be a simple questionnaire inquiring as to why the patient is leaving.

Developing and implementing an internal marketing plan does not have to be expensive. It will take time, thought, and commitment from everyone in the practice, however.

Tips

Drug companies are often willing to fund various aspects of your marketing program. Also, many hospitals now have physician practice enhancement centers to provide guidance, services, and funds to physicians who wish to develop marketing plans.

I suggest that you purchase *The Medical Marketer's Guide* published by the Medical Group Management Association [(303) 753-1111]. This inexpensive, excellent book is crammed full of practical information about all facets of practice marketing. It is an excellent starting point from which to launch your marketing plans.

LESSON 4–3: TASTEFULLY SPREADING THE WORD

I have been taking my laundry to the same dry cleaner for several years. The employees know my name, the service is always prompt and friendly, and they do a good job with my clothes. I discovered this dry cleaner through a direct marketing flyer that I received in the mail. If this business had not made the effort to contact me, I never would have discovered them, no matter how good they were.

This is external marketing.

If internal marketing is every action that you and your staff take to maintain the good will of your existing patients and referral sources, then external marketing is every action that you and your staff take to attract new patients and referral sources.

It is impossible to discuss external marketing without bringing up the dreaded "A" word: advertising. It is unfortunate that lawyers introduced the public to professional advertising. Who doesn't cringe when they see a television commercial with an attorney standing at the scene of an auto accident asking, "Have you had an accident? Call me. I can turn it into a check for you." Put that image aside for a moment and remember that not all advertising is done through the medium of television and that not all television ads are in poor taste.

The reason to consider external marketing, perhaps even advertising, is that when done properly it can be a most effective method of building your practice's market share. External marketing also effectively informs patients and fellow practitioners about programs or services in which your practice specializes.

The major disadvantage of external marketing is expense. External marketing usually requires that you hire a marketing/public relations specialist. Good ones are expensive. You also will have to commit practice dollars over an extended period of time to penetrate your market properly.

Of course, there are no guarantees. An excellent external marketing plan can only attract patients and referral sources. Your internal marketing plan has to be up to the task of keeping them. That is why it is important to remember that marketing is a continual process.

There are two keys to successful external marketing plans. First, it is imperative that you identify your target markets. An external marketing plan designed to reach patients differs from a plan that targets referring physicians, large employers, managed care plans, or specific demographic groups. Second, have a clear concept of the messages you want to communicate. What is the general message you want to convey to your target groups? Do you have specific messages, such as information about a niche or specialty that sets your practice apart? Be clear and concise.

Once you have identified your practice's target market and message, there are several mediums available to you to get the word out. All mediums should be discussed with your marketing people to determine which are best for your practice. Among the many marketing tools that you may wish to consider are the following:

- pure advertising
  1. newspapers
  2. magazines
  3. radio
  4. television
  5. telephone directories
  6. neighborhood direct mailers
  7. billboards
- free public relations

Cultivate a rapport with local print, radio, and television editors by issuing news releases and media kits about your practice. Register with a speakers bureau. Your goal is to be included in feature articles, health industry publications, radio and television talk shows, health fairs, and local magazines and newspapers.

Keep in touch with all physician referral sources, and take them to lunch or dinner periodically. Be available. Acknowledge their accomplishments with a call or a short letter. Communicate quickly with them about patients whom they have referred to you. Send holiday presents. Refer to them when the opportunity arises.

Again, certain aspects of external marketing can be expensive. I urge you to talk to drug companies and hospitals about offsetting part of the costs.

Finally, be patient. External marketing usually takes longer to bear fruit than internal marketing. Therefore, you must develop a plan in which you have confidence, hire experienced consultants, and then persevere.

LESSON 4–4: MARKETING IN A NUTSHELL

A well-developed, expertly implemented marketing plan is an indispensable practice management tool. Successful medical practices of the future will view tasteful marketing as an inherent part of practicing medicine. Practices that begin to develop a long-term marketing plan now will find themselves light years ahead of their colleagues in the competitive marketplace. The following checklist will help you begin the process:

1. The first step is for everyone in your practice to make a commitment to excellence in medicine.
2. Interview several marketing/public relations firms with experience in medical marketing. Review their work, and check their references. Select the firm that not only demonstrates its talent but also gives you the distinct impression that the success of your practice is important to them.
3. Determine your target markets.
4. Define the specific messages that you want conveyed to your target groups.
5. Develop an internal marketing plan.
6. Develop an external marketing plan.
7. Develop expectations by which you can judge the success of your internal and external marketing plans.
8. Have regular meetings to review, monitor, and adjust marketing plans.
9. Make the marketing process an integral part of your medical practice.

◆ Chapter 5 ◆

The Staff Management Short Course

LESSON 5-1: NO PHYSICIAN IS AN ISLAND

Recently I was involved in a struggle with a wasp nest situated on the second story of my home. The wasps won.

I fell off a ladder and tore cartilage and a ligament in my knee. After talking to several of my clients, I selected an orthopedic surgeon who came highly recommended. I made an appointment to see him and proceeded to wait in his office for two hours.

I asked his staff what was going on and was told that he was running late. I had pretty much already figured that out on my own. I complained. The receptionist rolled her eyes and told me that the physician was always late, as if this was a sufficient explanation. The nurse also was uninterested in my condition or my long wait. She refused to answer any of my questions and reminded me that she was not the physician. I had pretty much been able to conclude this on my own, too.

The surgeon finally showed up, quickly examined my knee, and told me I needed surgery and when he could perform the procedure. When I told him I wanted a local anesthetic, he said that he didn't perform arthroscopic surgery that way. Although this physician came highly recommended, I decided to seek a second opinion.

The second surgeon also was late for our appointment, but his staff were magnificent. They apologized, explained why he was late, and emphasized that this seldom happened. They asked whether I needed to use their telephone to inform anybody that I would be running late. They kept me updated about the physician's anticipated arrival and genuinely seemed to care about me as a potential patient. The nurse even listened to my wasp story (although why she found humor in it escapes me).

When the physician came into the room the first words out of his mouth were, "I'm really sorry to be running so late." He listened to my story, examined me, and let me ask questions. When I asked for a local anesthetic he said, "We can do you one better. We'll let you watch the whole operation on television and give you a videotape to take home."

Which physician do you think I selected?

Both physicians had equivalent surgical skills. The second physician, however, and particularly his staff, communicated a clear message to me: "We care about your medical condition, your concerns, and your time."

The practice of medicine today is high pressure, high tech, fast paced, and competitive. Physicians caught in the midst of this environment must never lose sight of this:

◆ **MEDICAL PRACTICE MANAGEMENT TRUTH 9** ◆

The most valuable asset in your practice is your employees.

You would think that this statement is nothing more than common sense. Several years ago, I thought so too. In 80% of the practices with which I consult, however, I hear serious staff complaints about how the physicians treat them. These are actual quotes:

"There is no organization here. I don't know who to ask questions."
"No one trains you. I don't know exactly what it is that I'm responsible for and who I'm responsible to."
"Hiring and firing are done too impulsively. I don't know where I stand. We never get any feedback."
"There is no consistency or uniformity in the application of the ever changing rules."
"The patients are treated like stars, but we get no respect. It is as if we don't have faces."
"Just when we get things organized, a doctor's spouse will come in and stir everything up worse than ever."

Your staff are the extra eyes, ears, mouths, hands, and feet you need to get everything accomplished. They bill, collect, keep the books, market, nurse, soothe, cater, and cover for you. They are human beings who need to be trained, encouraged, listened to, raised, promoted, and reviewed. Like most people, they will learn more from what they experience than from what they are told. If you treat your staff with respect and concern, they will treat your patients in the same manner.

The purpose of this chapter is to acquaint you with the basics of staff management. The following lessons will deal with screening and hiring, staff training, firing, promotion and compensation reviews, and policies and procedures manuals.

There is no substitute for having well-trained, enthusiastic, and motivated staff supporting your practice. If you have such staff, they will make your professional life, no matter how intense the stresses, like heaven. If you don't . . . well, you know.

LESSON 5–2: IF YOU THINK COMPETENT PEOPLE ARE EXPENSIVE, TRY HIRING INCOMPETENTS

Few occurrences are more disruptive to a medical practice than employee turnover. Losing a good employee is always unsettling. The subsequent interviewing, hiring, and training are time consuming and expensive.

The purpose of this lesson will be to discuss staffing requirements, recruitment sources, interview techniques, orientation, and training.

At our firm, the hiring process is kept in perspective by one Golden Rule: Always hire the absolute best people for a job, and pay them a salary that will keep them happy.

As a general rule, we pay our employees at least 10% above the market rate for their job. What does this accomplish? Simply put, we are able to attract and maintain the best talent available. More to the point, the higher the caliber of employees we hire, the easier our life is.

Staffing Requirements

Determining your staffing requirements is the beginning of the personnel process.

There are several books that can provide guidance on the number and types of staff whom each medical specialty needs. The *Cost and Production Survey Report,* published by the Medical Group Management Association, is one such book. For instance, it reveals that the average cardiology practice will need 3.6 full-time employees per physician. Many publications will also break this information down by job classifications such as bookkeepers, receptionists, nurses, and technicians. The truth is that common sense and discussions with your colleagues will give you an excellent idea of how large your staff should be.

Here are a few rules to guide you in staffing your practice:

- Prepare written job descriptions for each position. These job descriptions should be written by the employee, reviewed by you, and updated every year. A typical job description will outline duties to be performed and related deadlines. It also will outline who supervises this position and who is supervised in the position. New employees can use written job descriptions rapidly to gain a basic understanding of what will be expected of them. *The Group Practice Job Description Handbook,* also published by the Medical Group Management Association, is an excellent reference work on preparing job descriptions. It provides more than 250 sample job descriptions for more than 140 positions and a host of other valuable information.
- Do not mold a practice around the employees. This is a problem usually found in older, more established practices. Generally, one employee has not performed satisfactorily for

a long time but has been with the practice for so many years that the physician hates to let him or her go. The practice is now molded around this person's deficiencies. As a result, the practice must hire an additional employee to compensate. This causes two problems: increased payroll expense, and staff resentment.

- Strive to surround yourself with competence.

Recruitment Sources

There are several good techniques for locating new employees.

- *Word of mouth.* The grapevine is an effective, inexpensive way of getting the word out that your practice is seeking to hire an excellent employee.
- *Tell your staff.* Discuss the job requirements with them. Ask them to keep their eyes and ears open for a high-caliber individual who may be interested. You might offer a small bonus for locating an excellent individual who is ultimately hired. Another reason to inform your present staff about job openings is that one of them may be interested in filling the position. Promoting from within your organization is an excellent idea if the candidate has the aptitude for the new position.
- *Tell your colleagues.* You would be surprised at how many people approach physicians looking for job opportunities. For instance, an excellent hospital employee may be tired of long hours or shift work. He or she may have asked your colleague about a job, but there were no openings at that practice. Your colleague could pass along news of your opening.
- *Ask your consultants.* Your CPA may know a good bookkeeper looking for a job. Drug company representatives may know of laboratory technicians. A good practice consultant may know insurance clerks or administrators looking to change jobs. Get your consultants to spread the word for you.
- *Be creative in your search process.* An allergist gave me his secret for hiring good receptionists. While he was shopping with his wife, he noticed that many retail salespeople were excellent at dealing with the public. He knew they worked long hours for low pay. When he has an opening, he observes the salespeople and asks bright, friendly ones if they would be interested in interviewing with him.
- *Newspaper advertisements are OK at best.* The key to getting good results from newspaper ads is to ask for resumes to be sent to your office. Don't accept telephone calls. Screen the resumes, check references, and select a handful of the best applicants to interview.
- *Recruitment firms are generally a disappointment.* Despite their fancy brochures and promises to screen applicants closely, I find that they keep throwing people at a job opening until you hire one of them. These firms are also expensive.

Interview Techniques

The interview is one of the most important steps in the hiring process. It is unpleasant to have to terminate a new employee who isn't working out. A conscientious interviewing process can help prevent this from happening.

Your office manager should screen applicants, conduct initial interviews, and select the top two or three applicants for an interview with the physician. If your practice is large, one physician should be designated to oversee the process. Another approach is to have the physician with whom the employee will be working conduct the final interview.

The office manager and the physician should openly discuss candidates. Don't compromise your standards and hire someone out of frustration. Continue the interviewing process until you believe that you have identified a candidate who will bring excellence to the job.

Interviews should be summarized in writing. Exhibit 5–1 is a sample interview and evaluation checklist.

Orientation

Once you have hired a new employee, do more than show him or her to a desk. Make new employees feel important and welcome. Take time to tell them how much you are looking forward to working with them. Assign a big brother or big sister for a couple of days to teach them about the practice. Give new employees a tour of the office, and tell them where the supplies are and how to use office equipment. Introduce them to the rest of the staff, and review the policies and procedures manual with them.

Don't let a new employee eat lunch alone the first day on the job.

Training

The first training provided to new employees should, of course, be on-the-job training, augmented by in-service training programs. I recommend using outside experts periodically to enhance new employee skills. Even the best CPT coder can learn something new. So can your bookkeeper, office manager, technician, and receptionist.

The small amount of money you spend to bring in experts or to send your employees to continuing education courses will be quickly recouped. Fresh ideas will constantly flow through the practice, and employees will be honored that you thought enough of them to care about developing their skills.

Exhibit 5–1 Interview and Evaluation Checklist

Name of Potential Hiree: ____________________ Position Sought: ____________________

INSTRUCTIONS: This form is required to be completed in stages beginning with the initial interview of a potential hiree for a position on our office staff. The interviewer is responsible for completing Sections I, II, and III. The owner is responsible for completing Sections IV and V. Specific instructions are included under each section.

SECTION I—INITIAL INTERVIEW

Date of Initial Interview: ____________________ Location: _____ Office

Interviewer: ____________________ _____ Other (Specify)

A. Optional procedure: List any important questions you plan to ask the interviewee during the interview. (Attach additional pages if necessary.)

	Question	*Interviewee's Answers*
1.	____________________	____________________
	____________________	____________________
2.	____________________	____________________
	____________________	____________________
3.	____________________	____________________
	____________________	____________________
4.	____________________	____________________
	____________________	____________________
5.	____________________	____________________
	____________________	____________________

B. At the appropriate time during the interview, communicate the following firm policies that apply to the position sought by the candidate.

- advancement and performance review
- overtime
- reimbursement of job-related expenses
- vacation
- benefits
- ____________________
- ____________________
- ____________________
- ____________________
- ____________________

C. Circle the choice that best corresponds to the assessment of the candidate's potential that you reach during the interview.

Key: 5—Outstanding, 4—Above Average, 3—Average, 2—Below Average, 1—Not Acceptable, U—Unable to Evaluate.

1. Appearance. Did the candidate present a professional appearance? 5 4 3 2 1 U
2. Education. Does the candidate's educational background appear to be adequate for the position sought? 5 4 3 2 1 U

Exhibit 5–1 continued

3. Work Experience. Does the candidate's prior work experience appear to indicate the ability to assume responsibility and work well with other people? 5 4 3 2 1 U
4. Personality. Did the candidate display a desirable personality and friendliness? 5 4 3 2 1 U
5. Maturity and Judgment. Did the candidate appear to possess maturity and sound judgment? 5 4 3 2 1 U
6. Communication. Did the candidate express his or her ideas and thoughts in a concise, articulate manner? 5 4 3 2 1 U
7. Poise and Self-Confidence. Did the candidate appear poised and self-confident? 5 4 3 2 1 U
8. Attitude and Enthusiasm. Was an appropriate attitude and level of enthusiasm displayed? 5 4 3 2 1 U
9. Employment Objectives. Do the candidate's employment objectives appear to be compatible with the position sought, particularly as they relate to salary, benefits, responsibility, and overtime? 5 4 3 2 1 U
10. Quality of Responses. Were the responses to questions indicative of careful thought and sincerity? 5 4 3 2 1 U

OTHER COMMENTS: ____

____

____

____

____

____

Recommendation: ❑ Consider Employing ❑ Decline Offer

SECTION II—OTHER INFORMATION

Check additional information that you have requested from the candidate and attach that information to this form when obtained.

- ❑ Employment Application
- ❑ College or High School Transcript
- ❑ Resume
- ❑ References
- ❑ Recommendation Letters
- ❑ Other (specify) ______________________

SECTION III—REFERENCE CHECK

Indicate whether you desire that references be checked:

❑ Waive reference check.

❑ Please check references.

Exhibit 5–1 continued

	Reference 1	Reference 2	Reference 3
1. Date of inquiry.			
2. Person making inquiry.			
3. Name of prior employer or reference.			
4. Phone number.			
5. Position held.			
6. Salary.			
7. Duties and responsibilities.			
8. Would prior employer rehire applicant?			
9. Did applicant work well with others?			
10. Was the applicant well-received by patients with whom he/she came in contact?			
11. Does the applicant exhibit initiative and an ability to work with minimal supervision?			
12. Does prior employer believe applicant has necessary skills for position?			
13. Does prior employer have concerns about applicant's honesty and integrity?			
14. Is the applicant proficient with personal computers, data processors, or other office machines?			

SECTION IV—SUMMARY

❑ No offer made. (File this form in rejected offer file.)
❑ Employment offer made.
Date of offer: ______________________ Planned starting date: ____________
Starting salary and benefits: ______________________________
____
____
Approved by: ______________________________

SECTION V—FOLLOW UP IF OFFER IS MADE

❑ Offer Accepted. (File form in personnel file.)
❑ Offer Rejected. (File in rejected offer file.)

Source: Reprinted from *Guide to Physicians and Other Health Care Professionals* with permission of Practitioners Publishing Company, © 1990.

LESSON 5-3: A WORD ABOUT THE BAD EGG

Every medical practice has a bad egg from time to time: the hiring mistake, the employee who just does not fulfill expectations, the employee whose performance has grown progressively worse.

A brief lesson for handling terminations is therefore necessary: Terminate employees who need to go, do it with respect, and do it quickly.

This may sound insensitive. It isn't meant to be. Occasionally our firm has had to terminate an employee, and after all these years it has never gotten easier.

We all weave part of our ego, self-esteem, and sense of worth into our jobs. When someone tells us our performance is not good enough, it can be emotionally devastating. That is why handling the situation with respect for the individual who is being terminated is so important. Never take away an employee's dignity.

In spite of all of this, my experience still tells me to be direct for the following reasons:

- Attempts to salvage an employee gone bad seldom work.
- Lingering dismissals only prolong the agony for everyone.
- Good employees resent those who do not carry their share of the work load. Morale suffers.

When I work with smaller practices, I try to interview each employee. I always ask the employees to describe five practice strengths and weaknesses based on their own observations. Fellow employees taking advantage of the practice are listed as weaknesses over and over again. Your employees know who is not performing. It strikes a raw nerve with them. They might not say anything to you, but they know, and they don't like it.

Finally, employees who are not performing up to par are expensive in terms of payroll and in terms of alienating or even endangering patients. They cost money in receivables that don't get collected and insurance forms that don't get filed. Poor job performance hurts your practice's overall performance in a hundred ways.

When all is said and done, terminate them, do it with respect, and do it quickly.

LESSON 5–4: WON'T SOMEBODY TELL ME HOW I AM DOING?

I was a brand new, very green lieutenant in the Marine Corps during the Vietnam War. In my platoon I had a rebellious, streetwise kid from the ghetto who had an uncanny ability to avoid responsibility. Worse yet, by Marine Corps standards he was a slob.

I was on Private Mason day and night: "Shine your shoes, get a haircut, shave better, do it over until it's right." Of course, Private Mason only grew worse at everything he attempted.

One day as I was lamenting about Private Mason to a wise old gunny sergeant, he interrupted me in midcomplaint and said, "Sir, spend today finding things to tell the boy he's good at."

So I did. It wasn't easy, but I did. Private Mason began to change before my eyes.

Then one morning it happened. Private Mason fell out for roll call perfectly squared away, shoes shined, hair cut, uniform starched, standing tall, and looking proud. I called him to the front and announced, "Gentlemen, this is Private Mason. This is what the Marine Corps expects all of us to look like." Private Mason almost burst with pride. Soon thereafter, he was promoted and began to take on leadership responsibilities.

I will never forget the lesson the old gunny and Private Mason taught the know-it-all lieutenant about the power of positive feedback.

Earlier in this chapter I told you that a major complaint I hear from medical practice employees is that they never get any feedback. Physicians are often just too busy to see them as individuals. Yet every employee needs feedback. Employees want to know how they are performing. They need to hear that they are pleasing you and meeting your expectations. Periodically, someone has to tell them what they are doing well, what they need to work on, and what their job holds for them in the future.

On the other hand, I know that time is a precious commodity for you. So over the years I have developed a simple two-step employee evaluation process that works well in medical practices.

Step 1: The Formal Evaluation

Every June 30th, you and/or your office manager should meet individually with each employee and give him or her a formal written evaluation (if your practice is large, you may use the employee's anniversary date instead of June 30th for this meeting to spread reviews out over the year).

The *Guide to Physicians and Other Health Care Professionals,* published by Practitioners Publishing Company, has an excellent employee evaluation form (reproduced in Exhibit 5–2). You may customize this form to meet the needs of your practice, but certain basics should remain.

Exhibit 5–2 Employee Evaluation Form

Name: ______________________ Position: ______________________

Reviewed by: ______________________ Date: ______________________

INSTRUCTIONS: This evaluation should be made at least annually and should be based on performance since the last evaluation. After familiarizing yourself with the descriptions of ratings given below, indicate for each item the rating you consider most appropriate. The reviewer may want to mention specific strengths, weaknesses, or add general comments and suggestions to illustrate or explain any ratings given. Please note that GOOD is the typical or normal rating describing completely satisfactory work. Copies of this form should be furnished to the person being reviewed by the reviewer.

For each of the items listed, rate performance from OUTSTANDING to NOT APPLICABLE by placing a check in the appropriate space. Refer to the following description in assigning ratings:

Outstanding	indicates extraordinarily high performance, well beyond that expected of someone at this level.
Very Good	indicates performance that exceeds usual expectations of someone at this level.
Good	indicates performance that meets that expected of someone at this level.
Below Normal	indicates that assignments and responsibilities are not being met as well as expected.
Unacceptable	indicates unacceptable performance in need of immediate improvement.
Not Applicable	assignments during the evaluation period did not allow a proper evaluation of this attribute.

	Outstanding	Very Good	Good	Below Normal	Unacceptable	Not Applicable
1. Personal characteristics reflect a high degree of integrity, maturity, dependability, and enthusiasm.	___	___	___	___	___	___
2. Exercises good work habits to effectively perform assigned duties.	___	___	___	___	___	___
3. Keeps physician or immediate supervisor informed as of status of projects or problems that arise in routine duties.	___	___	___	___	___	___
4. Readily accepts responsibility and exerts efforts beyond demands.	___	___	___	___	___	___
5. Works with minimal supervision.	___	___	___	___	___	___
6. Respects confidentiality of not only patient information, but of certain administrative information as well.	___	___	___	___	___	___

Exhibit 5–2 continued

	Outstanding	Very Good	Good	Below Normal	Unacceptable	Not Applicable
7. Understands and adheres to office policy and procedures and internal office routines.	___	___	___	___	___	___
8. Is courteous, tactful, and cooperative with others in the office, recognizing the importance of teamwork.	___	___	___	___	___	___
9. Maintains a positive attitude.	___	___	___	___	___	___
10. Is loyal and projects a good image of the office.	___	___	___	___	___	___
11. Is well-received by patients.	___	___	___	___	___	___
12. Is receptive to criticism.	___	___	___	___	___	___
13. Is sensitive to appearance of the office.	___	___	___	___	___	___
14. Communicates effectively.	___	___	___	___	___	___

15. Strong points: ______________________________

16. Weaknesses: ______________________________

17. Suggestions/Comments: ______________________________

______________________ ______________________

(Date) (Signature)

ANNUAL PROMOTION AND COMPENSATION SUMMARY

Name of person evaluated: ______________________

Position: ______________________

Period of evaluation: ______________________

Strengths: ______________________

Exhibit 5–2 continued

____

____

Weaknesses: ____

____

____

____

____

Other comments: ____

____

____

____

____

Overall Evaluation: ____Outstanding ____Very Good ____Average ____Below Expectations
Prior year salary: ____
Recommended new salary: ______________________________________
Approved by: _________________________Date Approved: ______________

Source: Reprinted from *Guide to Physicians and Other Health Care Professionals* with permission of Practitioners Publishing Company, © 1990.

Discuss in specific terms employee strengths and weaknesses such as attitude, appearance, work product, ability to accept responsibility, and need for supervision.

Ask the employee how weaknesses can be improved in the upcoming year. Write the information down and then read it back, asking whether the employee understands it correctly. Have the employee review and sign the evaluation form.

This formal evaluation also is the time for annual raises. Yes, annual. Employees must understand that annual raises will be awarded based on two criteria. The first is how well they have performed their job, and the second is how well the practice has performed financially during the year.

The practice should strive to give raises that at least equal the annual rate of inflation. Employees who don't merit an inflation raise probably should not be working for the practice. On the other hand, if they do deserve a raise don't make them ask for it. A scheduled annual review lets all employees know when they are up for their next raise.

During the review, let the conversation be a two-way dialog. Encourage the employee to ask questions, make suggestions, and air complaints.

Exhibit 5–3, the staff salary review, should be prepared annually. This important document will give you a clear picture of total employee costs and a basis from which you can determine annual raises.

Exhibit 5–3 Staff Salary Review, December 31, 199X

Employee	199X Actual Salary	Hourly Rate	Hire Date	Ins.	Matching FICA	Pension	ETO* Days	Special Assessment	St/Fed Unemploy.	Total Compensation	Benefits as % of Base Salary
	$14,093	$7.50	02/17/92	$1,200	$1,078	$____	12	$197	$63	$16,643	18
	9,729	6.25	04/13/92	1,200	744	____	12	136	63	11,884	22
	40,174	19.00	06/20/88	1,200	3,073	3,499	18	210	63	48,219	20
	24,411	11.93	10/08/84	5,716	1,867	2,126	18	210	63	34,393	40
	12,480 (2)	6.00	01/18/93	1,200	954	____	12	174	63	14,871	19
	17,999	8.51	11/15/74	2,363	1,376	1,567	18	210	63	23,578	30
	16,233	8.26	10/03/88	2,363	1,241	1,414	16	210	63	21,524	32
	14,752	7.26	01/27/88	2,363	1,128	1,285	16	206	63	19,797	34
	10,345	4.25	10/01/91	1,200	791	____	16	210	63	12,609	21
	15,134	6.75	08/28/89	1,200	1,157	1,318	16	210	63	19,082	26
	13,061	6.78	12/28/88	2,363	999	1,137	18	182	63	17,805	36
	15,410	7.58	09/30/91	2,363	1,178	____	16	210	63	19,224	24
	16,678	8.32	05/22/89	1,200	1,275	1,464	16	210	63	20,890	25
	21,060	9.85	02/17/86	5,280	1,611	1,834	18	210	63	30,058	42
	11,923	6.50	02/03/92	1,200	912	____	16	167	63	14,265	19
	17,025	7.78	04/12/82	1,800	1,302	1,483	18	210	63	21,883	28
	32,103	14.90	07/27/87	1,800	2,455	2,796	18	210	63	39,420	23
	7,134	8.79	08/26/82	1,200	545	____	16	99	53	9,031	26
	17,238	7.75	03/16/92	1,200	1,318	____	12	210	63	20,029	16
	16,505	7.34	06/17/85	1,200	1,262	1,437	18	210	63	20,677	25
	15,698	7.15	08/17/81	1,200	1,200	1,379	18	210	63	19,750	26
	23,693	10.90	09/02/75	1,200	1,812	2,063	18	210	63	29,041	22
	13,718	6.46	02/03/86	1,200	1,049	____	16	192	63	16,222	18
	15,582	7.25	01/02/90	2,363	1,192	1,357	16	210	63	20,767	33
	62,495	29.27	12/28/89	5,716	4,207	5,842	18	210	63	78,533	26

*Earned time off (vacation and sick days, etc).

Step 2: The Informal Review

During December, you and/or your office manager should meet with each employee for a less formal review. During this meeting, the June 30th employee evaluation should be updated with notes about how the employee's performance has been for the last six months. (If you have a very large practice, this second meeting may not be practical.)

At this time, it may be appropriate to distribute a small holiday bonus depending on the customs of your practice. Generally, a bonus at this time is only a gift and should not be based on performance.

Summary

The two-step employee review process has several advantages:

- Employees receive formal feedback about their performance at least semiannually.
- Employees know when they will be reviewed for raises and don't have to work up the courage to ask for one or harbor anger over not knowing when one is coming.
- Communication is vastly improved. The practice now has an organized means of discussing employees' strengths and weaknesses and setting goals. Employees also have an opportunity to discuss any topics of interest to them.

The two-step review is a formal process. It is not meant to take the place of good day-to-day management of your personnel. Nothing can replace your noticing and telling employees about a job well done or how much you appreciate how they went out of their way to help a patient.

Physicians should continually reward good employees' performance. Give them an afternoon off when things are slow, buy your staff lunch, or send the office flowers. If you think that positive feedback isn't important . . . well, you have never met Private Mason.

LESSON 5–5: "THERE, UNDER THAT PILE OF DUST. ISN'T THAT OUR POLICIES AND PROCEDURES MANUAL?"

I am impressed by the number of practices that actually have policies and procedures manuals, big fat ones that must have cost a fortune. I am dismayed by the number of employees who never read them or know they exist. Your practice needs a viable policies and procedures manual that is periodically updated for accuracy and reviewed with your employees. At a minimum, the manual should:

- be custom tailored to your practice
- introduce employees to the practice and its philosophy
- give a brief history of the practice and its management
- discuss patient relations
- discuss internal policies
- explain employee benefits

New employees should be instructed to read the policies and procedures manual. Allow them to ask any questions they may have. In many firms employees are then required to sign a simple statement that they have read and understand the manual. Every so often, your practice should give an in-service class on the policies and procedures manual. This class should remind employees of key practice policies, especially those that have changed since they were hired.

An excellent reference source for drafting your practice's policies and procedures manual is *The Group Practice Personnel Policies Manual,* published by the Medical Group Managers Association.

LESSON 5–6: LOOKING FOR THE LEADER

A bad medical office manager can wreck your practice.

Two recent consulting engagements brought this point home to me quite clearly. Recently, I was contacted by a large cardiology group that had a vague notion that something was wrong with their practice. The practice was expanding rapidly, they were constantly hiring new physicians, and everybody was busy, but physician incomes were dropping significantly.

As usual, I requested a great deal of documentation to begin the practice management review. The first indication of a problem was that the office manager could not provide much of the documentation requested. The information she was able to give showed serious accounts receivable problems. The entire process of coding, billing, and collections was out of control, very seriously so. Additionally, expenses were growing geometrically.

As I began my practice management review and started to dig deeper and deeper, I discovered that virtually every practice management problem known to humanity existed in this practice. It was in many ways the same old story: excellent physicians trying to keep up with the demands of geometric patient growth and leaving the management of their business to the office manager. The office manager started with the practice when it was small and did not have the skills necessary to manage its explosive growth. Overwhelmed, she lived in denial, attributing the problems to resource-based relative value scales or insignificant excuses such as spending too much money on snacks for employees. When confronted with page after page of serious problems, she shrugged her shoulders and started to rattle off the typical excuses: "It's not my job, I don't have enough time, we don't do it that way here, I didn't know that." The cost of bad management? Conservatively, I estimate that this practice has lost $500,000 to $750,000 per year for at least the last three years. This is a significant amount of money even to this large practice.

I also consulted with a urology practice that had virtually the same problems. At one time this group was dominant in their city. Trouble began when they brought in a new office manager with little medical experience and few management skills. In a very short period of time collections began to drop, expenses began to increase, staff morale hit rock bottom, and the physicians were at each others' throats. Once we began to unravel the tangle, it became clear that all the threads were leading back to an inept office manager. The cost to this group was approximately $150,000 per year in lost collections.

Loss of dollars and cents is not always the most serious loss, however. If an incompetent office manager allows you continually to bill Medicare incorrectly, you may be confronted with significant legal problems far more alarming than lost collections. Bad managers also cost a practice by causing staff turnover, by hiring low-caliber employees who pose no threat to them, and by making the place where you spend most of your waking hours miserable.

Historically medicine has been practiced through a multitude of small practices. Often when physicians started out, they hired a new staff. The person who stayed the longest eventually became office manager by virtue of seniority.

Now, all of a sudden medicine is big business, and group practices typically gross several million dollars a year. I would guess that there is no other field where so many million-dollar corporations are run by high school graduates who learned their trade on the job. Medical office management is a complex profession to learn. These are just a few of the skills a competent office manager needs to master:

- personnel management
- patient education and patient relations
- appointment scheduling
- billing, coding, and insurance processing
- dealing with all aspects of managed care
- computer systems
- financial analysis and management
- internal and external marketing basics
- medical record maintenance
- dealing with agencies such as the Occupational Safety and Health Administration, Medicare, the Department of Labor, and so forth
- quality assurance issues
- strategic planning
- providing specialty services
- dealing with physicians
- the ability to lead, manage, and motivate staff

Attaining excellence in office management is not easy.

How can you tell whether your office manager is doing a good job? Look and listen. Does your office manager have information readily available, or do you always have to go see so-and-so to find what you are looking for? Are problems always blamed on someone else? Is it hard to determine exactly what your office manager does? Does it seem that most of his or her time is spent on routine matters that should be delegated to others? Does your office manager spend time with the staff, asking questions, teaching, and making sure that everything is going smoothly, or does he or she hole up in the office? Are there a lot of long lunches, sick days, or days when the manager leaves early? Do you have a sense that your practice is headed in the wrong direction and that all you hear are excuses? Is there a lot of staff turnover? Does the office manager seem to surround himself or herself with poor-quality staff? Any combination of the wrong answers to these questions may indicate that your manager is in over his or her head. Don't bury yours in the sand.

Over the next decade you will see medical practice management evolving into a true profession. There will be many more degreed and well-trained people available to manage the complexities of medical practices. Right now, however, much of the responsibility for hiring and training the right office manager depends on you, the physician. Here are some helpful hints:

- Hire excellence. Do not settle for someone who is only adequate because you are in a hurry to hire or because you don't want to pay the salary that excellence requires. One way or another, you will pay the price. The person you hire doesn't necessarily have to have a strong medical background, although it helps a great deal. It is essential that you hire an intelligent self-starter who can quickly learn what he or she needs to know. This person must keep his or her skills sharp as well as lead, motivate, and train your staff. He or she also must be diplomatic and polished enough to handle physicians, patients, and staff with ease.
- Train your office manager. Few people will come to your practice with all the skills listed above. Your office manager should attend at least two continuing education courses (that you pay for) a year. Dollars spent to keep your office manager on the cutting edge of what is happening in the field will be repaid to you many times over. I also would insist that the office manager join the Medical Group Management Association.
- Set expectations. You should communicate clear, concise expectations to your office manager. Everyone needs structure and goals to stay focused not only on the task at hand but also on the bigger picture. Expectations will aid the manager in moving the practice in the direction you want it to go.
- Make the office manager accountable. The manager must report regularly to a person or group. This accounting will compare the expectations placed on the office manager with his or her actual performance. With an excellent office manager, this will be a team meeting, a time when all management meets to ask: "Where are we now?" "Where are we going?" "What is the best way to get there?"
- You, the physician, must stay involved with your office manager. Never delegate complete authority to run the practice. Even the best office managers may go astray if you do not play an active role in the management of your practice.

LESSON 5–7: STAFF MANAGEMENT IN A NUTSHELL

Your employees are essential to your practice's smooth operation and financial success. Too often, they are taken for granted. Ignored employees get discouraged and perform below their capabilities or look for better employment elsewhere. Here are 10 steps to help you convey the message to each of your employees that "you are the backbone of my practice, and I truly appreciate your efforts on my behalf":

1. Hire the right number of employees for your specialty and size. Don't hire too many employees, but don't try to cut corners by hiring too few.
2. Conduct in-depth interviews to fill job openings.
3. Hire only the best people.
4. Pay top wages.
5. Train your employees well, and encourage them to keep up with the latest developments in their field.
6. Meet with your employees at least semiannually, and give them formal written performance evaluations.
7. Give periodic raises, bonuses, and performance rewards.
8. Develop and use your policies and procedures manual.
9. When necessary, terminate nonperforming employees quickly.
10. Talk to your staff, encourage them, and show them that you care about them and their careers.

◆ Chapter 6 ◆

The Short Course on Advisors

LESSON 6–1: BEWARE OF THE FIRM HANDSHAKE AND THE BIG SMILE

The Bible sums it up best: "Plans fail for lack of counsel, but with many advisers they succeed" (Proverbs 15:22).*

In these perplexing times, you must rely on the wisdom and advice of several professionals to deal with all the complexities of your business and personal finances. The problem, then, is to discern which are wise counselors and which are charlatans. The price for not knowing can often be disaster.

Each of us has at least one friend who has lost a significant amount of money by acting on poor advice from a so-called professional. I speak with at least one physician a month who has lost money in this way. What amazes me is how people who have worked so hard and so long to accumulate money can so easily turn that money over to a near stranger to manage it for them. Seldom are references checked, contracts read, investments researched, or the

---

*Taken from the HOLY BIBLE, NEW INTERNATIONAL VERSION, copyright 1973, 1978 by the International Bible Society, used by permission of Zondervan Bible Publishers.

"smell test" applied. The reason is usually the same: "He was such a nice guy and seemed to know what he was talking about."

Before we discuss specific types of advisors, there are a few general rules that apply to dealing with all of them.

Rule 1: You Can't Just Delegate and Walk Away

A good personality, articulate speech, a firm handshake, and a big smile are no guarantee of competency. In representing my clients over the years I have met with some of the most polished and impressive incompetents and crooks that you could ever imagine.

The simple fact is this: You must always stay involved. No one, not even the wisest and best-intentioned counselor in the country, will ever care about you and your family's financial situation as much as you should. Counselors should offer wise advice, but you must do your homework to understand each situation thoroughly and make your own final decisions.

Rule 2: Build a Team

If you check references and do your homework, you will be able to compose a team of advisors who will help you navigate through life. At minimum, your team should consist of an excellent attorney, a CPA, an insurance agent, a banker, and perhaps a stockbroker. You may have to go through several of each before you find the best.

Rule 3: Pay the Price

There is a story about a man who found himself in the middle of a serious, potentially expensive problem. He hired the best lawyer available to deal with it. A few days later the lawyer called his client and told him that, through his contacts, he had been able to correct the problem.

The man was greatly relieved until the end of the month, when he received a large invoice from the attorney. Irate, the man called his attorney, demanding to know how he could charge so much for only a few days' work. The lawyer answered, "Gunslingers don't charge by the bullet." Good advice is expensive, but compared with what bad advice may cost, it is indeed a bargain.

The purpose of this chapter is to acquaint you with the advisors with whom you will ultimately have to deal throughout your career. These advisors generally fall into two distinct categories. The first category of advisors comprises those who charge by the hour or provide financial assistance as part of their job. Examples are attorneys, CPAs, and bankers. Those in the second category work on a commission basis. Examples include insurance agents, stockbrokers, and some financial planners.

With a little work, you will easily be able to compile a list of advisors who are technically excellent in each of their respective fields. Technical proficiency isn't enough, however. What you are really seeking in an advisor is wisdom, common sense, honesty, and loyalty.

Take time to interview the people on your list. Ask yourself whether this is a person with whom to build a lifetime business relationship. Will this person tell me what he or she thinks I want to hear or what I need to hear? Does he or she really care about my situation? Is he or she technically excellent in his or her field? When you can answer yes to these questions, you have found someone to serve on an advisory team for life.

LESSON 6–2: IT'S ALL THE SAME TO ME, I'M PAID BY THE HOUR

I am prepared to take a lot of criticism regarding my advice about using advisors. My opinions are based on years of observing who and what works and who and what does not. These are general statements to which there are certainly exceptions. If my advice is wrong based on your personal experience, so be it. If I save you from making an expensive mistake because of a misplaced trust, however, I feel that I have done my job.

The first group of advisors we'll discuss comprises those paid by the hour or paid by someone else to be available to you. This lesson will discuss the educational background, training, and practice methods for CPAs, attorneys, and bankers. It also will address selecting, using, and developing a relationship with these professionals.

CPAs

To practice as a CPA, an individual usually must have the following minimum requirements:

- a bachelor's degree in accounting
- successful completion of a 3-day national examination that covers topics such as accounting practice and theory, auditing, taxation, and business law
- in most states, a 1- to 2-year apprenticeship before being fully licensed
- fulfillment of the mandatory continuing education requirements of the state in which the CPA is licensed to practice

CPAs will usually choose an area of specialization, such as auditing or taxes, early in their careers. Although they are not allowed to hold themselves out as specialists, it is common practice for CPAs to specialize in certain industries. You will want to make sure that your CPA has an in-depth understanding of medical practices.

CPA firms range in size from solo practitioners to large international firms. Generally, large firms are primarily interested in large corporate clients and are not suited to delivering the personalized services medical practices need. Local or regional CPA firms are much more likely to have expertise in medical practices and to regard them as first-class clients.

The best way to choose the CPA who is right for you is to get references from your fellow physicians or from a trusted advisor, such as your banker or attorney. Select two or three CPAs who come highly recommended, and interview them.

Don't be afraid to ask questions; it is important to get a feel for how it will be to work with this individual for many years to come. At the end of the interview, ask for the names and numbers of three physicians who have been the CPA's clients for several years. Call these physicians, and ask them how extensively they use the CPA and how satisfied they are.

Make sure you discuss fees. CPAs charge by the hour, with fees typically ranging from $60 to more than $200 per hour depending on the size of the firm and its particular expertise in an area. Find out in advance what hourly rate you will be charged and approximately how much your annual fees will be. A CPA should be happy to provide this information to you in an engagement letter. Exhibit 6–1 is a detailed example of an engagement letter customized for work to be performed for a large medical group.

CPAs are generally conservative in the advice they render. Because they charge by the hour, they also tend to be objective and frank. If a deal is rotten, your CPA is likely to tell you so.

What you don't want in a CPA is a form-filler-outer. You also do not want your practice to be a training ground for your CPA firm's new accountants. Make sure that the CPA firm you engage understands that you expect experienced individuals working on your account.

Your CPA should be familiar with the medical field and should be willing to help you analyze your practice and develop and implement creative solutions to practice problems.

If you have general questions regarding CPAs, the American Institute of Certified Public Accountants, (212) 596-6200, can answer them; it also keeps records of who has passed the CPA examination. State boards of accountancy can inform you about any disciplinary actions taken against licensed CPAs.

Here are some specific questions that you might ask the CPAs whom you are considering engaging:

- Tell me about your present medical clients and the experience your firm has in the health care field.
- How will you staff my account?
- How accessible will the partner on my account be, and how involved will he or she get in analyzing our corporate financial data and aiding in making management decisions?
- How does your firm charge for its services? What can I expect my first year fees to be?
- Does your firm administer corporate pension plans?
- Does your firm coordinate, as necessary, overall decision making among the professional corporation, the corporate pension plan, and the physician's personal financial situations?
- Will you provide us with a reference list of several of your physician clients?
- How quickly can we expect to receive financial statements and tax returns that your firm prepares? Will you review them in detail and on a timely basis with us?
- Where do you see health care headed in the next 10 years?
- What type of specialized health care services does your firm provide? Examples might be:
    1. complete practice evaluations
    2. CPT coding reviews
    3. new practice set-ups

Exhibit 6–1 Sample Engagement Letter

Dear Dr. ———:

This letter is to confirm our understanding of the terms and objectives of our engagement and the nature and limitations of the services we will provide.

We will perform the following services for (company):

1. Compile from information you provide the monthly statement of assets and liabilities–tax basis and the related statement of revenue and expenses–tax basis. We will not audit or review such financial statements. Our report on the monthly financial statements is presently expected to read as follows:

   We have compiled the accompanying statement of assets and liabilities–tax basis of (company) as of (date) and the related statement of revenues and expenses–tax basis for the year then ended, in accordance with standards established by the American Institute of Certified Public Accountants. The financial statements have been prepared on the tax basis of accounting, which is a comprehensive basis of accounting other than generally accepted accounting principles.

   A compilation is limited to presenting in the form of financial statements information that is the representation of management. We have not audited or reviewed the accompanying financial statements and, accordingly, do not express an opinion or any other form of assurance on them.

   Management has elected to omit substantially all the disclosures required by generally accepted accounting principles. If the omitted disclosures were included in the financial statements, they might influence the user's conclusions about the company's financial condition. Accordingly, these financial statements are not designed for those who are not informed about such matters. If, for any reason, we are unable to complete the compilation of your financial statements, we will not issue a report on such statements as a result of this engagement.
2. Prepare the federal and state income tax returns for the above named company for its appropriate year end.
3. Aid you in your administration of a pension plan, preparing, as needed, annual tax filings, participant statements, summary annual reports, and trust accountings.
4. Prepare federal and state individual income tax returns for the physicians (and their children) of (company).
5. Attend your bimonthly meetings and present a management report.
6. Prepare necessary payroll tax returns.
7. Develop and aid the corporation in monitoring internal accounting controls.
8. Develop a management information system that establishes goals, monitors them, and places specific expectations on key employees.
9. Provide sundry business discussions, phone calls, and the like.

Our engagement cannot be relied upon to disclose errors, irregularities, or illegal acts, including fraud or defalcations, that may exist. We will inform you of such matters that come to our attention, however.

We will provide the services above for 1 year at $XXXX/month beginning (date). This fee includes travel expense.

In addition to the above, we will complete the following one-time projects over the next 12 months:

1. Accounts receivable management: The management of accounts receivable would initially require staff training in coding systems (ie, CPT, HCPCS, ICD-9, evaluation and management, and modifiers), redesign of hospital and office superbills, restructuring of fee schedules, staff training in computer management capabilities, and design of daily, weekly, and monthly collections policies and procedures. Additionally, formal and fiscally responsible policies for adjustments and write-offs, past due accounts, and insurance claims follow-up need to be redesigned for optimal reimbursement. Once these policies are implemented, accounts receivable management would include continuous monitoring for procedure compliance, problem solving, crisis management, and attainable goal setting to reduce the size of the total accounts receivables and to shift the weighted percentages from having greater than 50% past–120 days to greater than 50% pre–90 days.

Total estimated hours over 12 months	300 hours
2. Fee schedule analysis	20 hours
3. Medical records quality control system implemented	20 hours
4. Risk management systems implemented	20 hours
5. Coding reimbursement policies	20 hours
6. Staff training	30 hours

These projects will require approximately 400 hours of staff time. We will spend no more time on a project than is absolutely necessary. Our fees are as follows: partners, $115–$145 per hour; consultants, $100 per hour; accountants, $65–$90 per hour; clerical, $55 per hour. Additionally, we will invoice you for basic travel expenses at our cost. Project work will be billed on a separate monthly invoice. Payment of our invoices is due and payable within thirty (30) days of the date of our statement.

Your returns are of course subject to review by the taxing authorities. Any items resolved against you by the examining agent are subject to certain rights of appeal. In the event of examination, we will be available to represent you and will bill you for additional services at our standard rates for them.

We shall be pleased to discuss this letter with you at any time.

If the foregoing is in accordance with your understanding, please sign in the space provided and return this letter to us.

Sincerely,

Robert W. Katz
Katz & Asher, Ltd

RWK/rhl
Acknowledged:

______________________________ ______________________________
(Physician) Date

4. contract negotiations with health maintenance organizations (HMOs), preferred provider organizations (PPOs), hospitals, and the like
5. medical practice evaluations
6. physician buy-in/buy-out assistance
7. reimbursement analysis
8. fee schedule reviews
9. superbill review and design
10. practice consolidations
11. physician retirement planning
12. receivables review/clean-up
13. embezzlement control analysis.

Attorneys

I have a great deal of respect for attorneys. The majority of attorneys with whom I have worked over the years have impressed me as competent advocates for their clients. Many also have been excellent counselors, a precious quality you should seek in your attorney.

In most states, attorneys must have a bachelor's degree and a law degree. They must have passed a tough state examination to earn a license to practice. Many states now require that attorneys complete a stipulated number of continuing education hours each year.

Like CPAs, attorneys practice in firms ranging in size from one person to several hundred lawyers. Attorneys tend to be highly specialized. Your best bet is to find an attorney who specializes in the health care industry with extensive business and taxation experience. So much the better if the attorney has a master's degree in tax law.

Once again, the best way to select an attorney is through referrals from physicians or trusted advisors. Interview several attorneys, and ask questions. Make sure that they have extensive experience with professional corporations and medical practices. Your attorney also should be able to provide wise counsel in estate and tax planning, wills and trusts, pension plans, general business contracts, and, of course, resolving business disputes.

Discuss fees. Legal research and document drafting can be time consuming. You should reach a clear understanding of costs before engaging your attorney for projects. Your attorney's advice should be objective, conservative, and professional. Again, you are looking for a relationship with a lifetime counselor. Keep searching until you find it.

You can inquire of your state's bar association as to disciplinary action taken against any of its licensed attorneys.

Here are some specific questions that you may wish to ask attorneys whom you are considering engaging:

- What experience does he or she have with:
  1. dealing with third party reimbursement entities such as HMOs, PPOs, insurance companies, and related government agencies?
  2. antidumping laws (eg, Combined Omnibus Reimbursement Act)?
  3. safe-harbor laws and related self-referral problems?
  4. contractual arrangements between physicians and hospitals?
  5. accounts receivable collection laws?
  6. professional corporation and limited liability entity laws?
  7. real estate law?
  8. labor and employment law?
  9. medical malpractice and quality assurance issues?
  10. general business, tax, and estate planning laws?
- What experience does the lawyer have in representing physicians within your particular specialty?
- Will the attorney provide you with a list of other physician clients for reference checking purposes?
- What are the attorney's standard fees for professional services? How much should you expect to pay on an annual basis? (Depending on the size of your corporation, you should expect to pay at least $1,000 to $5,000 per year in legal fees.)
- Who will actually be working on your account? How accessible will the partner on your account be?
- What can the attorney do to ensure that you are kept informed of changes in health law, labor law, and so forth that affect your practice? Will he or she be proactive?

Bankers

It is always a good idea to establish a relationship with at least one bank. During the last 10 years the banking world has become highly competitive. As a result of this competition, banks have established executive and professional departments (sometimes called private banking departments) designed specifically to attract and cater to professionals.

These departments make the bank a more friendly place for you. They will help you manage your cash flow, provide favorable loan terms, cut through red tape, and offer general counsel on a variety of business matters. Find out whether your bank has such a department and what services it offers.

You should meet with your bank officer a couple of times a year to update him or her on your business and personal finances. Maintaining a personal relationship with your banker speeds up the process when you need the bank's help.

A good banker also should be a good sounding board. Bankers are usually objective and conservative and may provide you with an interesting point of view on an investment you may be considering. Generally, bankers will not be as familiar with medical practices as your CPA or attorney, yet good ones offer sound business advice, and the price is right.

Here is a list of questions that you may ask the officers of the private banking department that you are considering using:

- Can I access all your bank's services through you?
- Do you have an investment advisor in your department? (Although banks are prohibited by law from selling securities, many private banking departments still have investment advisors on their staffs.)
- How available will my private banking officer be? Will there be a back-up when he or she is out of the office? (A major complaint from physicians relates to high turnover in private banking departments.)
- What products and services does the department offer (eg, loans, money market accounts, and checking accounts)?
- How financially stable is the bank? Will you provide us with copies of the bank's financial statements?
- What services can you provide, such as authority verification, to help our group reduce the opportunities for fraud?
- What is your knowledge and experience with health care clients?
- Do you have a background in and offer both consumer and commercial loans?
- Can you provide me with a list of references to check?
- What services and/or training can you provide for my staff? How can you help me make the medical practice operate more efficiently?
- Do you have the authority to approve most of my borrowing needs?
- Talk to me about service. What does that mean to you? (For instance, I would expect a willingness on the bank officer's part to come to your office to transact business.)
- What are your fees for the various services the bank offers?
- Where are your branch offices located?

LESSON 6–3: I'M ON COMMISSION, AND I LOVE YOU

The next group of advisors—insurance agents, stockbrokers, and financial planners—works on commission. Every time you deal with one of these individuals, a red light should go off in your head, and you should hear the words: If he doesn't sell me something, he doesn't eat.

Now understand, there are lots of excellent insurance agents and stockbrokers, and there are a few good financial planners, but there are an awful lot of marginal and bad ones as well. As a general rule, this group of professions should be viewed first as salespeople and secondarily as advisors.

No one does more financial harm to my clients than commissioned advisors. So even though you need them, you also need to be careful in selecting and using them.

Insurance Agents

If attorneys are not as bad as everyone thinks they are, insurance agents are not as good as they would have you believe. I say this after many years of practice, repeatedly observing that, no matter what the financial problem, buying a life insurance policy seems to be the insurance agent's standard solution. I can only assume that the high commissions associated with certain life insurance policies somehow factor into the agent's advice.

Becoming an insurance agent does not require a college degree, and virtually anyone can become licensed to sell life insurance. Therefore, obtaining referrals and checking references are important when you select an agent.

It is even more important that you check out the stability of the insurance company that is underwriting the particular insurance policy that your agent is selling. Insurance agents come and go, but you may have to rely on your insurance company for 30 or 40 years. Make sure that the company is financially sound. Chapter 8 contains information about how to obtain ratings on insurance companies. You can call the National Association of Insurance Commissioners, (816) 842-3600, to obtain the phone number of your state's commissioner of insurance. This office can be helpful in providing you with information about insurance companies and agents in your state.

Also, many magazines, such as *Consumer Reports* and *Money*, periodically have issues that rate insurance companies based on their financial stability, quality of their policies, and quality of claims service.

Buying life and disability insurance will have financial implications for your life for years to come. These are not decisions to be taken lightly or to be based on how friendly an agent may be. Investigate before you invest. What should you look for in an insurance agent? I'll tell you what I looked for and found in my agent. First, he represents only high-quality insurance companies. The information he provides me makes common sense and is presented professionally, in detail, and without pressure. Over time, he has demonstrated that he is truly concerned about the aspects of my financial plan that he represents. He knows his limitations.

If you do not have the time or the desire to perform the necessary analysis of proposed insurance policies, let someone independent of the insurance agent do it for you. This individual should be able to analyze your insurance needs and find the policies that best satisfy those needs. (Insurance will be discussed further in Chapter 8.)

Stockbrokers

If you are a physician, you will be called by a different stockbroker about once a month for the rest of your life. This may be partially due to the fact that it is easy to obtain a securities license.

Stockbrokers used to sell only equity products, such as stocks and bonds. Now most large brokerage firms have expanded to offer additional products such as mutual funds, pension plans, certificates of deposit, credit cards, mortgages, and, yes, even life insurance.

Stockbrokers work for two different types of brokerage firms. Large, full-service firms such as Merrill Lynch or Smith Barney Shearson execute transactions, offer investment advice, and provide unending research, reports, and financial products. Discount brokerage firms, on the other hand, offer little or no research and advice, but they will buy and sell securities for you at a commission rate lower than the full-service firm's. All commissions are now negotiable. So even if you deal with a full-service brokerage firm, don't be afraid to ask for a discount if you trade frequently or deal in large dollar volume transactions.

The National Association of Securities Dealers, (301) 590-6500, maintains records on all registered brokers. These records keep track of federal and state actions against brokers. The Securities and Exchange Commission, (202) 272-7450, also keeps records on disciplinary actions taken against brokers and financial planners.

Because it is likely that a broker may handle a great deal of your money, it is important that you stay involved. Here are 10 rules for dealing with stockbrokers based on the mistakes I see most commonly:

1. Never, never give your broker discretion to trade in your account without your approval. You must understand and approve every investment that you make.
2. Balance your portfolio. Each investment should be evaluated in terms of safety, liquidity, and yield. Your portfolio should be well diversified and include stocks from a variety of industries, bonds with staggered maturity dates, and ample cash to see you through short-term emergencies.

3. Buy and hold your investments. Don't allow your account to be churned by constant buying and selling.
4. Stay away from high-commission proprietary products. Many brokerage firms package and sell their own mutual funds or limited partnerships. Generally, they have a high commission and perform poorly.
5. Never buy anything based on a cold call over the telephone.
6. Never buy penny stocks.
7. Never buy anything sold hard as a sure thing or sold with the warning, "If you wait, you'll miss out on tremendous profits."
8. Realize that your investments will not help you escape from your profession. I have never seen anyone make so much money in the stock market that he or she could dramatically change his or her life style.
9. Realize where your brokerage account fits in your overall financial picture (this will be discussed in more detail in Chapter 8).
10. Understand your broker's educational and professional background. How many financial decisions of high magnitude are you willing to delegate to a Russian history major?

Financial Planners

There are tens of thousands of people out there, everywhere, handing out cards that give them the dubious title of financial planner. Many are insurance agents and stockbrokers who use the title *financial planner* as an alias for their true identity.

The financial planning industry has no mandatory educational requirements and no effective regulatory body. This means that anyone can call himself or herself a financial planner, which is a potentially dangerous situation.

Financial planners usually provide services in one of two ways. The more reputable financial planners work on a flat fee basis and receive no commissions. If you are going to use a financial planner, this is the type that you should use. These people will meet with you on several occasions, familiarize themselves with your financial situation, and then prepare a financial plan for you. About 10% of all financial planners operate this way. A typical flat fee will be approximately $1,000 to $3,500, or 1% of monies managed.

The second kind of financial planner is commission-based. These people charge little or nothing for the financial plan, and they earn a living from the commissions they receive on the products that they sell. Of course, these products are the ones that they have already recommended to you in your financial plan.

My own (biased) opinion is that you should use your attorney and CPA to develop and monitor your financial plan. Generally, they are the best educated and qualified to do so.

Here are some questions that you may wish to ask if you are trying to select a financial planner:

- How does the planner get paid? The physician should expect a complete breakdown on all sources of income to the financial planner as well as an accounting of how much the planner made from his or her relationship with any companies for which he or she sells products.
- Is the planner a registered investment advisor? If yes, then request a copy of the planner's Securities and Exchange Commission's Form ADV. This document will allow you to review the education and training background of the planner and his or her staff.
- If the planner is not a registered investment advisor (this is likely, and therefore the planner is a product salesperson), then request a resume, including a listing of any and all product vendor contracts and agreements.
- What specifically will be included in the planner's financial plan? Request a copy of a sample plan.
- Ask the planner to provide references from other clients and professional people (lawyers and CPAs) with whom he or she works.
- How many years has the planner been in the financial planning field?
- What back-up staff and support people are available to assist you when the planner is not available?
- How many other clients does the planner have?
- What are the services the planner provides and the cost for each service?
- What type of liability insurance coverage does the planner carry? Who is the carrier? Ask to speak with the carrier.

LESSON 6–4: ADVISORS IN A NUTSHELL

To navigate the waters of today's complex society, you often must depend on the counsel and advice of CPAs, attorneys, insurance agents, and stockbrokers. So watch out.

To find the best advisors:

- Always check references. Ask colleagues for recommendations. Find out why they like a particular professional. Find other physicians who use a particular professional, and question them about his or her performance.
- Always interview the professional whom you are considering engaging. Try to get a feel for how you will work together. Does he or she look you straight in the eye? Are his or her answers to your questions clear and accurate, or does he or she circumvent your questions? Does he or she ask good questions?
- As soon as you suspect that advice may be inappropriate or incorrect, get a second opinion.
- Clearly understand the differences between fee-based and commission-based advisors, and act accordingly.

Remember that a true professional will understand that you are doing him or her a favor by being a client. If you are made to feel that the relationship is the other way around, find a new advisor.

INSERT

TAB

◆ Part II ◆

The Retirement Plan

◆ Chapter 7 ◆

The Retirement Short Course

LESSON 7–1: I HOPE YOU ARE NOT DEPENDING ON SOCIAL SECURITY

I've seen the following scenario far too often.

Across the desk from me sits a physician in his 50s who has earned a good living throughout his professional life. He had always planned to slow down about now to enjoy life.

The problem is that he has saved nothing. His salary has all gone to maintaining a very comfortable life style. He may even have significant debts. Now, just when he wants to slow down, his three children are about to enter college, and the reality of tuition, books, housing, and living expenses has staggered him. Any extra money he may have anticipated using for early retirement is sucked into the cost of higher education. At this point, many physicians find themselves remortgaging their homes just to meet new financial demands. It all becomes clear now: no early retirement, no slowing down, and questionable ability to retire at age 65.

Retirement planning is so important that I have given it a separate chapter rather than including it in the personal finance section of this book.

There are three keys to successful retirement planning:

1. *Fund early.* The sooner you begin to fund your retirement, the easier it will be for you to achieve your retirement goals.
2. *Fund annually.* Contribute to your pension plan every year without fail. A good rule of thumb is to try to put about 10% of your income (or up to $30,000 a year) into your plan.
3. *Don't play games.* Once you have put money into a retirement plan, invest it wisely. In fact, your retirement plan should be among your most conservative investments.

The remaining four lessons of this chapter discuss retirement planning and retirement plans in view of what is best for you, the physician. The lessons will answer these questions: How much money will you need to retire? What resources on which to retire should be available to you? What retirement plans are best for medical practices? What retirement plan pitfalls should you be wary of?

LESSON 7–2: SO, HOW MUCH IS ENOUGH?

Figure 7–1 illustrates how well you can expect to fare at retirement based on your preretirement income. If your retirement income is 0% to 50% of your preretirement income, you are in for a difficult retirement. You may have to change to a simpler lifestyle and continue to work part time. If your retirement income is 55% to 70% of your preretirement income, your retirement may be comfortable. A retirement income that is 80% or more of your preretirement income should put you in excellent financial shape to retire. Your goal now must be to start taking the necessary action to ensure that your retirement income is at least 70% of your preretirement income.

0%	50%		80%	100%
TROUBLE	FAIR	GOOD	EXCELLENT	

Figure 7–1 Retirement income as a percentage of your preretirement income.

LESSON 7–3: HOW TO GET THERE FROM HERE

Your retirement income will generally come from three major sources (Figure 7–2):

1. Your retirement plan
2. Your assets and their earnings
3. Social Security.

This lesson will discuss the income you can expect to receive from a retirement plan and from Social Security. Chapter 8 will discuss investment income.

Your Retirement Plan

Your retirement plan will more than likely be the greatest single source of income for your retirement. If your practice does not have one, I strongly urge you to adopt a pension plan as soon as possible. The best retirement plans for medical practices will be discussed in the next lesson.

Now, I want to impress you with the magic of compounding. Table 7–1 illustrates what a physician can accumulate by establishing a retirement plan and funding it with $20,000 a year while earning an 8% annual yield.

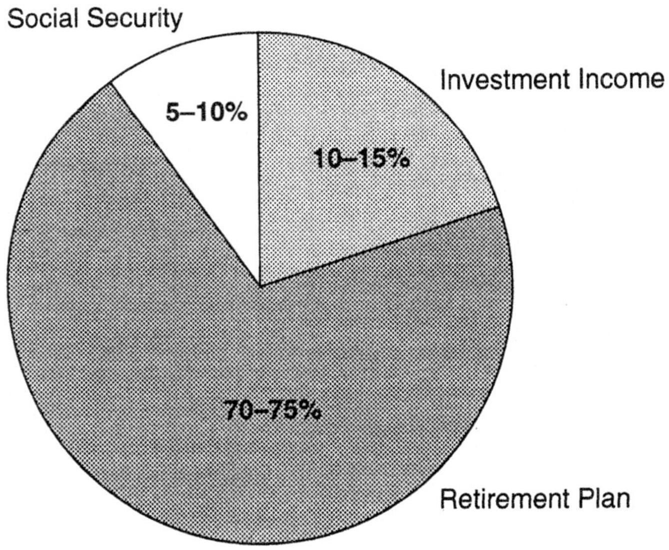

Figure 7–2 Income sources for retirement.

Table 7–1 Projected Pension Benefits

Age When Retirement Funding Begins	Amount Available at Age 60
30 years	$2,265,664
35 years	$1,462,119
40 years	$ 915,239
45 years	$ 543,042
50 years	$ 289,731
55 years	$ 117,332

What does this mean? The physician who started funding his or her plan when he or she was 30 will at age 60 be able to withdraw approximately $200,000 per year in retirement income for the next 30 years. Even after adjusting for inflation, this annual income should allow almost every physician to retire in comfort.

Unfortunately, the physician who waited until he or she was 50 to begin funding his or her pension plan can only withdraw about $25,000 per year starting at age 60.

Your retirement plan should provide at least 70% to 75% of your retirement needs.

◆ **MEDICAL PRACTICE MANAGEMENT TRUTH 10** ◆

In most cases, your ability or inability to retire will be directly related to how much you have accumulated in your pension plan.

Social Security

The Social Security system is actually three separate funds. The Disability Insurance Trust Fund pays benefits to disabled workers. A second fund, one with which you are probably all too familiar, is the Hospital Insurance Trust Fund, or Medicare. The third, and the one on which this lesson will concentrate, is the Old-Age and Survivors Insurance Trust Fund, which provides monthly checks to retirees, their families, and families of deceased workers.

Social Security was never intended to provide full retirement income. It was always intended to be only a supplement. Most physicians will find that it is a very small supplement. The largest benefit you can expect to receive in 1992 will be about $13,000. If you are 40 now, it is projected that you will receive approximately $17,000 per year when you reach age 65.

I often hear complaints along the lines of, "I don't know why I have to contribute to Social Security. By the time I am old enough to collect it, the system will be bankrupt." Bankrupt?

I doubt it. Since 1983 Social Security taxes have been raised tremendously, and the system now has a huge surplus of funds stockpiled in anticipation of the baby boomers reaching retirement age. This aging population will be a political force with which to reckon. Therefore, Social Security will not be abandoned by our concerned politicians.

The bad news is that there will probably be reductions in Social Security payouts, payout caps, increases in the minimum age to receive benefits, and increased taxation of benefits. The actual benefit you ultimately receive will depend on your age at the time you request benefits, how long you were in the workforce, and how much you contributed to the system.

To determine the present status of your Social Security account, you can call 1-800-772-1213 or go to the Social Security office and ask for form SSA-7004. It is a good idea for you or your CPA to check on your account every three years to verify that your earnings are being properly posted to your account.

The bottom line still remains: Don't rely heavily on Social Security to fund your retirement. Count on Social Security to meet only 5% to 10% of your retirement needs.

LESSON 7–4: THE BEST RETIREMENT PLANS FOR MEDICAL PRACTICES

There are several kinds of excellent retirement plans. It has been my experience that two types of plans are best suited for the majority of medical practices:

1. the profit-sharing plan (integrated with Social Security)
2. the money purchase plan (which also can be integrated with Social Security).

Exhibit 7–1 compares the general characteristics of every major type of pension plan.

The Profit-Sharing Plan

In the profit-sharing plan, my favorite for most medical practices, the practice, as employer, contributes toward each employee's pension account. This contribution is a percentage ranging from 0% to 15% of the employee's compensation. The contribution is strictly discretionary on the part of the employer. In good years the employer may choose to contribute a full 15% of employee compensation. If the employer has had a lean year, the contribution can be reduced or eliminated. All contributions made to the pension plan are tax deductible to the employer and nontaxable to the employee until they are withdrawn.

A profit-sharing plan has the following advantages:

- It is the most flexible of all pension plans. In good years the employer can make large contributions, but there is no obligation for the employer to make any contribution.
- This plan can be integrated with Social Security. This means that the employer, when calculating the contribution for employees, is allowed to take a calculated credit for the Social Security it has paid for employees. The net effect is to skew the contribution in favor of highly compensated employees, such as the physicians.
- It is the least expensive plan to set up. Many reputable brokerage firms have first-class prototype documents that an employer can adopt for a reasonable cost. One of the best profit-sharing plan prototypes that I have come across is offered by the brokerage firm A.G. Edwards & Sons, Inc. There are many good ones available. Two cautions when adopting prototypes: First, have someone who is familiar with prototypes review the one in which you are interested. You want to make sure that you adopt all the key provisions in a manner that is best for your practice. Second, make sure that you understand your ongoing responsibilities. You have to submit annual reports (form 5500 C/R) that a brokerage firm will not prepare. The responsibility for properly filing these reports lies with the physicians as trustees of the plan, and there are serious penalties for not complying.

Exhibit 7–1 Comparison of Employer Retirement Plans

Capabilities/ Restrictions	SEP-IRA *(Simplified Employee Pension)*	Salary Reduction SEP *(SR-SEP)*	Profit Sharing *(Defined Contribution)*	401(k) Profit Sharing *(Defined Contribution)*	Money Purchase *(Defined Contribution)*	Pension Plan *(Defined Benefit)*	403(b) Tax-Sheltered Annuities
Definition	A simplified employee pension is a plan through which employer contributions are made to IRAs established and maintained by eligible employees. These tax-deductible contributions must be allocated by the employer on a nondiscriminatory basis.	Plan for an employer with 25 or fewer eligible employees who can elect to make SEP contributions through salary reduction. Salary reduction agreement is combined with conventional SEP so that both employer and elective salary reduction employee contributions may be made.	Plan into which employer makes discretionary contributions on behalf of employees. All contributions plus earnings are allocated to individual accounts, which determine the individual's benefit at retirement. The formula for determining the amount of the employer's contribution may be fixed (such as a required percentage of profits or payroll), fully discretionary, or a combination of both.	Plan permits a cash or deferred arrangement as part of an employer's profit sharing or stock bonus plan. The arrangement is typically in the form of salary reduction between the employer and employee under which a contribution will be made only if the employee elects to reduce his compensation or forego a salary increase. Special nondiscrimination tests apply.	Plan has a definite contribution formula in which the employer promises to contribute a definite amount each year (such as a percentage of compensation or salary) on behalf of each participant. All contributions plus earnings are allocated to individual accounts, which determine the individual's benefit at retirement.	Plan is established so that the amount of the employee's retirement income is fixed, defining the benefit in advance by the plan's benefit formula. The employer's contribution must be determined actuarially and be sufficient to enable the fund to meet its liabilities as they come due in future years. Plan assets are not allocated to individuals' accounts.	Tax sheltered retirement program established by exempt employers and public education organizations for their employees. Plan may be funded on a non-discriminatory basis through salary reduction or deferral of salary increase. 403(b) account may only invest in annuities or mutual funds.
Obligation to Contribute	Employer makes voluntary contributions and can change each year or discontinue.	Salary reduction is voluntary; however, at least 50% of eligible employees must elect salary reduction. Some obligation for employer contributions to SEP if plan is top heavy.	Unless fixed as a percentage of compensation or profits, contributions are at the discretion of the employer and are not dependent on profits.	Contributions can come from voluntary employee salary reduction or from employer, or both. Employer may have some obligation to contribute if plan is top heavy.	Employer must meet minimum funding requirement. Percentage contribution chosen by the employer when plan is adopted must be met annually.	Employer must meet minimum funding requirements, dictated by the benefit formula and calculated annually by an actuary.	Contributions typically come from employee salary reduction. Employer contributions permitted, but may subject the plan to additional reporting/discrimination requirements.

Exhibit 7–1 continued

Maximum Deductible Contribution	Employer deduction cannot exceed lesser of 15% of participants' compensation or $30,000.[10]	Employer deduction limits are the same as SEP-IRAs. Employer contributions together with salary reduction cannot exceed the overall deduction limitations.[10] Salary reduction cannot exceed $8,994.[1]	Employer deduction cannot exceed 15% of aggregate participants' compensation. Allocation to each participant cannot exceed the lesser of 25% of compensation or $30,000.[9,10]	Employer deduction limits are the same as for profit sharing plans. Employer contributions together with salary reduction cannot exceed lesser of 25% of compensation or $30,000.[10] Salary reduction amount cannot exceed $8,994.[1]	Contributions cannot exceed the lesser of 25% of participant's compensation or $30,000.[10]	Amount needed to fund monthly benefit at normal retirement age. Annual benefit from the plan may not exceed the lesser of 100% of participant's compensation or $115,641.[1,2]	Maximum annual salary reduction is lesser of $9,500 or 20% of gross compensation. Employer contributions together with salary reduction cannot exceed lesser of 25% or $30,000.[10]
Prospects	Business owner who wants simplicity. Ideally suited for company with more volatile profits and low employee turnover.	Small employers who want to minimize employer contributions. Prospects also include employers with existing SEPs who want to add salary reduction feature.	Best suited for company with more volatile profits where employee turnover may be a problem. Usually better than money purchase if contribution rate does not exceed 15% of payroll. Usually better than SEP if company has part-time employees.	Best suited for company that wants to minimize employer contributions and encourage employee savings. Usually suited for larger companies because of cost of administering the plan.	Company with stable yearly profits (no problem contributing in good or bad years). May be useful in combination with profit-sharing plan.	Suited for established companies with consistent profits. Benefits companies with key employees over age 50.	Public schools or nonprofit organizations such as charitable or religious groups.
Entity or Person That Can Establish Plan	Corporation Partnership Self-Employed S Corporation Nonprofit	Corporation Partnership Self-Employed S Corporation	Corporation Partnership Self-Employed S Corporation Nonprofit	Corporation Partnership Self-Employed S Corporation	Corporation Partnership Self-Employed S Corporation Nonprofit	Corporation Partnership Self-Employed S Corporation Nonprofit	Educational Institutions Tax-Exempt 501(C)(3) Organization

Exhibit 7–1 continued

Capabilities/ Restrictions	SEP-IRA *(Simplified Employee Pension)*	Salary Reduction SEP *(SR-SEP)*	Profit Sharing *(Defined Contribution)*	401(k) Profit Sharing *(Defined Contribution)*	Money Purchase *(Defined Contribution)*	Pension Plan *(Defined Benefit)*	403(b) Tax-Sheltered Annuities
Eligibility	Includes all employees over age 21 who have worked for employer for any part of 3 of last 5 calendar years. May exclude employees earning less than $385 in the current year.[1]	Includes all employees over age 21 who have worked for employer for any part of 3 of last 5 calendar years. May exclude employees earning less than $385 in the current year.[1]	Possible exclusions: under age 21; employees who have worked less than 1,000 hours per year of service; less than 2 years of service.[3]	Possible exclusions: under age 21; employees who have worked less than 1,000 hours per year of service; less than 1 year of service.[3]	Possible exclusions: under age 21; employees who have worked less than 1,000 hours per year of service; less than 2 years of service.[3]	Possible exclusions: under age 21; employees who have worked less than 1,000 hours per year of service; less than 2 years of service.[3]	Employees of public schools or 501(C)(3) organizations.
Establishment/ Contribution Deadline	Must be established and contributions made by due date of employer's tax return, including extensions.	Must be established and employer contributions made by due date of employer's tax return, including extensions. Employee salary reduction contributions must be taken out of current compensation during the tax year.	Must be established by tax year end and contributions made by due date of employer's tax return, including extensions.	Must be established by tax year end and employer contributions made by due date of employer's tax return, including extensions. Employee salary reduction contributions must be taken out of current compensation during the tax year.	Must be established by tax year end and contributions made by due date of employer's tax return, including extensions.	Must be established by tax year end and contributions made by due date of employer's tax return, including extensions.	Can be established anytime during calendar year. Employee salary reduction contributions must be out of current compensation during the tax year. Employer contributions must be made by due date of employer's tax return, including extensions.
Can be Integrated With Social Security[4]	Prototype SEP—Yes. IRS model SEP—No.	Yes.	Yes.	Yes, if discrimination tests are met.	Yes.	Yes.	Yes.

Exhibit 7–1 continued

Vesting Requirements	Immediate 100%.	Immediate 100%.	Generally, plans must meet the following requirements: non-top heavy: 5-year cliff or 3- to 7-year graded; top heavy: 3-year cliff or 6-year graded.[4]	On employee elective deferrals, immediate 100%. On employer contributions, generally plans must meet the following requirements: non-top heavy: 5-year cliff or 3- to 7-year graded; top heavy: 3-year cliff or 6-year graded.[4]	Generally, plans must meet the following requirements: non-top heavy: 5-year cliff or 3- to 7-year graded; top heavy: 3-year cliff or 6-year graded.[4]	Generally, plans must meet the following requirements: non-top heavy: 5-year cliff or 3- to 7-year graded; top heavy: 3-year cliff or 6-year graded.[4]	Immediate 100%.
Minimum Contribution/ Benefit for Top-Heavy Plans	Up to 3% of compensation to all non-key employee participants.	Up to 3% of compensation to all non-key employee participants.	Up to 3% of compensation to all non-key employee participants.	Up to 3% of compensation to all non-key employee participants.	Up to 3% of compensation to all non-key employee participants.	Minimum benefit of lesser of 2% of compensation times years of service or 20% of average compensation for non-key employee participants.	Not applicable.
Taxation of Distributions	Ordinary income.	Ordinary income.	Pretax portion taxed as ordinary income. Pre-1974 contributions may be capital gains. Possible forward averaging for lump sums. Mandatory 20% withholding applies unless direct rollover transfer.	Pretax portion taxed as ordinary income. Pre-1974 contributions may be capital gains. Possible forward averaging for lump sums. Mandatory 20% withholding applies unless direct rollover transfer.	Pretax portion taxed as ordinary income. Pre-1974 contributions may be capital gains. Possible forward averaging for lump sums. Mandatory 20% withholding applies unless direct rollover transfer.	Monthly pension payments taxed as ordinary income. If lump sum, same as money purchase pension.	Ordinary income. Mandatory 20% withholding applies unless direct rollover transfer.

Exhibit 7–1 continued

Capabilities/ Restrictions	SEP-IRA *(Simplified Employee Pension)*	Salary Reduction SEP *(SR-SEP)*	Profit Sharing *(Defined Contribution)*	401(k) Profit Sharing *(Defined Contribution)*	Money Purchase *(Defined Contribution)*	Pension Plan *(Defined Benefit)*	403(b) Tax-Sheltered Annuities
Additional Taxes on Withdrawals Before Age 59½.[5]	10% penalty applies to withdrawals before age 59½ unless certain exceptions apply.	10% penalty applies to withdrawals before age 59½ unless certain exceptions apply.	10% penalty applies to withdrawals before age 59½ unless certain exceptions apply.	10% penalty applies to withdrawals before age 59½ unless certain exceptions apply.	10% penalty applies to withdrawals before age 59½ unless certain exceptions apply.	10% penalty applies to withdrawals before age 59½ unless certain exceptions apply.	10% penalty applies to withdrawals before age 59½ unless certain exceptions apply.
Requirements for Withdrawals After Age 70½.[6]	Mandatory annual distribution commences after age 70½. Minimum required distribution based on life expectancy.	Mandatory annual distribution commences after age 70½. Minimum required distribution based on life expectancy.	Mandatory annual distribution commences after age 70½. Minimum required distribution based on life expectancy.	Mandatory annual distribution commences after age 70½. Minimum required distribution based on life expectancy.	Mandatory annual distribution commences after age 70½. Minimum required distribution based on life expectancy.	Mandatory annual distribution commences after age 70½. Minimum required distribution based on life expectancy.	Mandatory annual distribution commences after age 70½. Minimum required distribution based on life expectancy. Generally applies to benefits accruing after 1986.
Loans[7]	Not allowed.	Not allowed.	Permitted if allowed by plan. See plan document for provisions.	Permitted if allowed by plan. See plan document for provisions.	Permitted if allowed by plan. See plan document for provisions.	Permitted if allowed by plan. See plan document for provisions.	Permitted if allowed by plan. See plan document for provisions.
What Happens When the Employee Leaves? (Forfeiture)	Unaffected by terminations.	Unaffected by terminations.	Forfeited funds may be reallocated among remaining participants, or may be used to reduce employer contributions.	Forfeited funds may be reallocated among remaining participants, or may be used to reduce employer contributions.	Forfeited funds may be reallocated among remaining participants, or may be used to reduce employer contribu-	Forfeited funds are used to reduce subsequent contributions.	Unaffected by terminations.

Exhibit 7–1 continued

Reporting and Disclosure	Minimal. Employer fills out SEP agreement and gives copy when employee becomes eligible.	Minimal. Employer fills out SEP agreement and salary reduction SEP agreement and gives copy when employee becomes eligible.	Full ERISA requirements. IRS Forms 5500, 5500-C, 5500-R or 5500-EZ annually.	Full ERISA requirements. IRS Forms 5500, 5500-C or 5500-R annually.	Full ERISA requirements. IRS Forms 5500, 5500-C, 5500-R or 5500-EZ annually.	Full ERISA requirements. IRS Forms 5500, 5500-C, 5500-R or 5500-EZ annually.	May require full ERISA requirements. IRS Forms 5500, 5500-C or 5500-R annually if employer makes contributions or is sufficiently involved.

[1] The limitation will be subject to cost of living adjustments in the future.

[2] May be actuarially adjusted if benefits begin before Social Security retirement age or if plan is not maintained for at least 10 years.

[3] Minimum coverage and participation rules apply.

[4] Top-heavy minimums apply when more than 60% of account balances/accrued benefits are attributable to key employees or in SR-SEP if key employee defers salary.

[5] In addition, 15% excise tax on large distributions may apply instead of 10% penalty.

[6] If the actual payment is less than the minimum required distribution, there is a 50% penalty tax on the difference.

[7] Certain loans to owner/employees or highly compensated employees may be prohibited transactions.

[8] Except for loans used to acquire a principal residence.

[9] Allocation refers to the total of employer deductible contributions, forfeitures and any employee salary deferral or voluntary after-tax contribution.

[10] Maximum compensation cannot exceed $235,840, adjusted annually for cost of living.

This summary is intended to be a brief overview of retirement plans and is incomplete. Specific situations should be referred to your tax or legal advisor.

Courtesy of A.G. Edwards & Sons, Inc., St. Louis, Missouri.

- A profit-sharing plan is the easiest plan to administer on an annual basis.
- It is the only plan you will ever need. If your practice establishes a profit-sharing plan early in your career and consistently funds that plan, it should provide all your retirement needs by age 60.

The only drawback to a profit-sharing plan is that, starting in 1994, the compensation ceiling used to calculate an employee's benefit decreases to $150,000 from the 1993 ceiling of $235,840. This means that, starting in 1994, the most that you will be able to contribute for any one employee is $22,500 (15% × $150,000).

The Money Purchase Retirement Plan

A money purchase pension plan is very similar to a profit-sharing plan except that it has a fixed contribution. For instance, the annual contribution required in the plan document may be 10% of every eligible employee's compensation. The employer is now obligated to make this annual contribution regardless of the practice's financial performance.

Because of this inflexibility, I only recommend money purchase plans under certain circumstances. The major advantage of a money purchase plan is that you are allowed to contribute as much as 25% of an employee's compensation (up to $30,000 a year). This is helpful when the physicians in a group know, without a doubt, that they want to contribute the maximum amount allowed under the law ($30,000).

With a profit-sharing plan, the most that can be contributed for any employee is $22,500. With a money purchase retirement plan, an employee can receive a $30,000 maximum annual contribution with a salary of only $120,000 ($120,000 times the 25% maximum percentage allowed for money purchase plans).

Although the money purchase plan allows you to contribute up to 10% more than a profit-sharing plan, I would be careful about making such a large commitment. A fixed plan should only be adopted by older physicians playing catch-up because they waited too long to adopt a plan.

An alternative is to adopt a money purchase plan in conjunction with a profit-sharing plan. For instance, your practice may have a money purchase plan that commits it to a fixed contribution of, say, 5% or 10% of salary per year and then a profit-sharing plan that allows for an additional discretionary contribution of up to 15%.

A Final Word

Keep it simple. For nine of every ten practices, a profit-sharing retirement plan integrated with Social Security will inexpensively satisfy all your retirement needs. I strongly recommend that you hire an expert, such as an attorney or CPA familiar with pension plans, to guide you through the process of adopting your retirement plan and to help you in its annual administration. You can expect to pay a one-time fee of between $500 to $2,000 initially to adopt your plan and $500 to $1,000 a year to have it professionally administered.

LESSON 7–5: RETIREMENT IN A NUTSHELL

Here are the five biggest problems that I encounter with medical practice retirement plans:

1. *No plan exists.* For most physicians, there is just no excuse for not adopting a retirement plan. The usual excuses I hear are, "I just don't have the money to put away right now," "Contributions for my employees are too expensive," and "I can save enough money on my own to retire on."

   Sorry, but these are just excuses. First, I have never been associated with a medical practice that could not afford a retirement plan if the physicians were committed to adopting one. Second, there are several methods of reducing the cost of employee pension contributions. One excellent technique is to integrate your plan with Social Security. Also, remember that a retirement plan is an excellent fringe benefit that will help you attract and hold on to the best employees. Finally, it is extremely difficult for anyone to save, on an after-tax basis, enough money for retirement.
2. *The plan is poorly funded.* Too often, a medical practice will come to the end of its fiscal year and find that there is little cash available for a pension contribution. The tendency then is to think, "I'll only contribute $5,000 this year, and I'll catch up in future years." That seldom happens. Make your pension contribution a monthly expense. At the beginning of each year, sit down with your advisors and establish a pension contribution goal. Divide that goal by 12, and contribute this amount into the pension plan monthly. By doing this, your plan will earn tax-deferred income on its assets sooner, and the practice will get into the good habit of properly funding the plan.
3. *The plan is poorly invested.* The funds in your pension plan must be wisely and conservatively invested. As a rule of thumb, I would keep 5% of the funds in a money market or short-term bond account, 45% to 50% in intermediate-term investment-grade bonds, and 45% to 50% in stocks. No-load mutual funds are an excellent way to attain this diversified portfolio. Don't try to pick market tops and bottoms. Your pension investments are long-term, and generally you should buy and hold them. Be patient with the normal stock market and interest rate cycles. Remember, your goal is to earn an average return of 9% to 12% on your pension assets. This goal does not require taking large risks in speculative investments.

   Exhibit 7–2 compares the historical rates of returns for portfolios with various stock-to-bond ratios. For instance, a pension portfolio that was 50% stock and 50% bonds would have had an average annual yield of 9.3% over a 42-year period. In its worst year the portfolio would have lost 11.1%, and in its best year it would have gained 31.6%.

   There is a rule of thumb that by subtracting your present age from 100 you will be able to determine the percentage of your long-term investments that should be invested in stocks. For example, if you are 45 years old you should have 55% of your long-term assets invested in stocks. The theory is that you should take a more aggressive investment position if you do not need the money for many years; then, as you get closer to retirement, you should gradually become more conservative. I cannot argue with this logic, but I believe that each physician should closely review Exhibit 7–2 and determine his or her individual comfort level.

A tip: Be careful about letting a bank trust department manage your pension assets. It has been my experience that the typical physician's pension account is too small for the bank, although the bank will never admit it. The accounts are often neglected, and the return is often poor.

4. *The physician plays games with the plan.*
   - Don't put money into your plan and then borrow it out.
   - Don't buy life insurance in your plan.
   - Don't buy limited partnerships, collectibles, or any of a dozen other highly speculative and ridiculous investments.
   - Don't make loans to friends and associates with plan assets.
5. *Details are not attended to.* The annual administration of your retirement plan must be completed properly and on a timely basis. Pay particular attention to the plan's tax return (Exhibit 7–3). If this form is not filed on time, the penalties can be onerous: $25 a day up to a maximum of $15,000. Make sure your CPA, attorney, or pension administrator has been assigned, in writing, the task of complying with all pension plan reporting requirements.

Exhibit 7–2 Finding Your Center: Risk Versus Reward

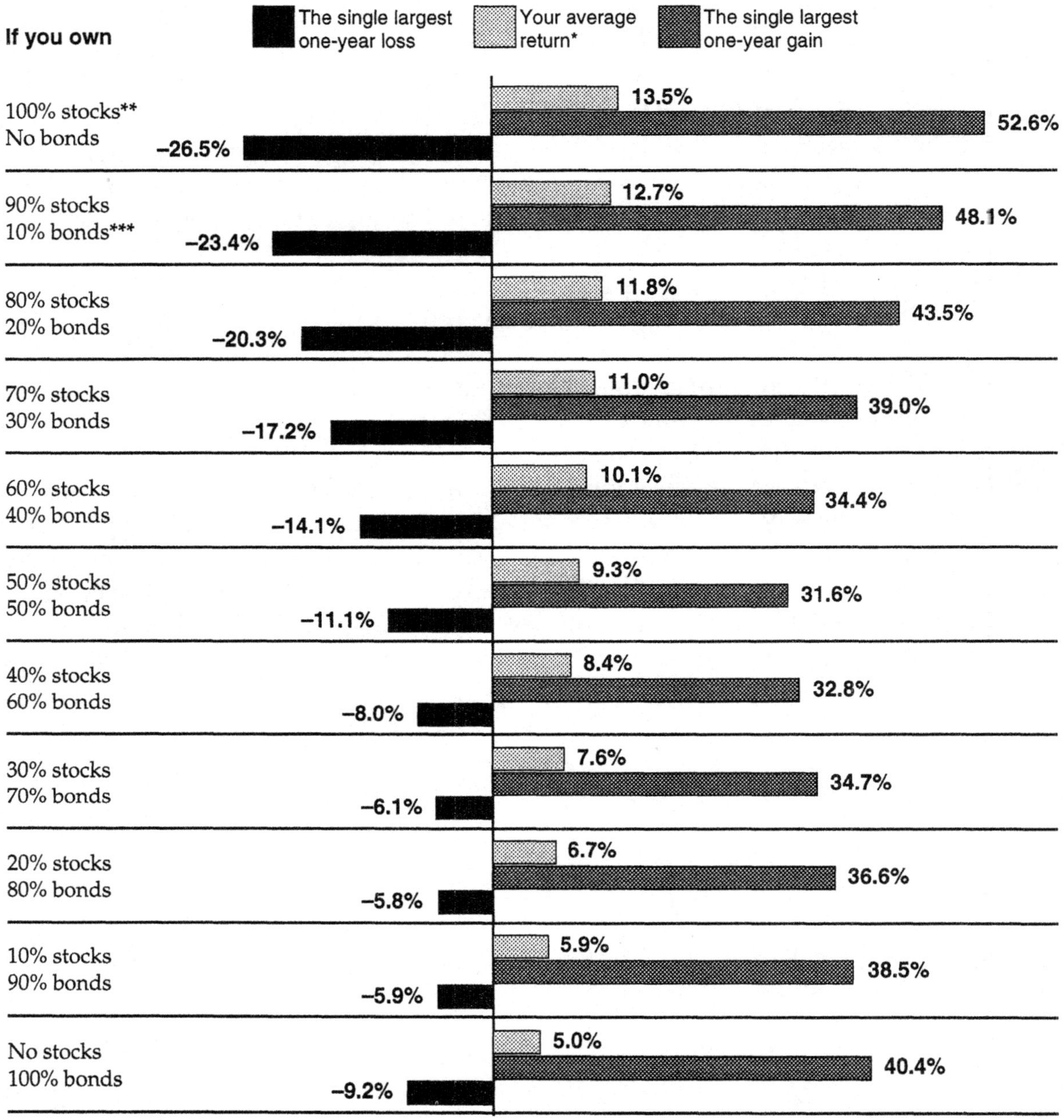

* From 1947–1989, compounded annually, dividends reinvested.
** Measured by Standard & Poor 500.
*** Long-term U.S. government bonds.
Sources: Towneley Capital Management, New York: Standard & Poor's Corporation; Ibbotson Associates; Crandall, Pierce and Company.
Courtesy of Bornstein Design Group, North Miami Beach, Florida.

Exhibit 7–3 Retirement Plan Tax Return

Form **5500-C/R**
Department of the Treasury
Internal Revenue Service
Department of Labor
Pension and Welfare Benefits Administration
Pension Benefit Guaranty Corporation

Return/Report of Employee Benefit Plan

(With fewer than 100 participants)

This form is required to be filed under sections 104 and 4065 of the Employee Retirement Income Security Act of 1974 and sections 6039D, 6047(e), 6057(b), and 6058(a) of the Internal Revenue Code, referred to as the Code.
▶ See separate instructions.

OMB No. 1210-0016
1992
This Form is Open to Public Inspection.

For the calendar plan year 1992 or fiscal plan year beginning , 1992, and ending , 19

You must check either box (5) or (6), whichever is applicable. See instructions.

For IRS Use Only
EP-ID

A If *(1)* through *(4)* do not apply to this year's return/report, leave the boxes unmarked. This return/report is:

(1) ☐ the first return/report filed for the plan;
(2) ☐ an amended return/report;
(3) ☐ the final return/report filed for the plan; or
(4) ☐ a short plan year return/report (less than 12 months).

(5) **Form 5500-C filer check here** . . . . ☐
(Complete only pages 1 and 3 through 6.) (Code section 6039D filers see instructions on page 6.)
(6) **Form 5500-R filer check here** . . . . ☐
(Complete only pages 1 and 2. Detach pages 3 through 6 before filing.) If you checked box *(1)* or *(3)*, you must file a Form 5500-C. (See page 6 of the instructions.)

If the preprinted information in 1a through 6d is incorrect, please correct it; if any information is missing, please add it. Be sure to include this page with your completed return/report.

B IF YOU CORRECT ANY OF THE PREPRINTED INFORMATION OR ADD MISSING INFORMATION IN 1a THROUGH 6d, CHECK HERE ▶ ☐
C If your plan year changed since the last return/report, check here . . . . ▶ ☐
D If you filed for an extension of time to file this return/report, check here and attach a copy of the approved extension . . . . . ▶ ☐

1a Name and address of plan sponsor (employer, if for a single-employer plan) (Address should include room or suite no.)

1b Employer identification number

1c Sponsor's telephone number

1d Business code (see instructions, page 19)

1e CUSIP issuer number

2a Name and address of plan administrator (if same as plan sponsor, enter "Same")

2b Administrator's employer identification no.

2c Administrator's telephone number

3 If you are filing this page without the preprinted historical plan information and the name, address, and EIN of the plan sponsor or plan administrator has changed since the last return/report filed for this plan, enter the information from the last return/report in 3a and/or 3b and complete 3c.

a Sponsor .... EIN .... Plan number ....
b Administrator .... EIN ....
c If 3a indicates a change in the sponsor's name, address, and EIN, is this a change in sponsorship only? (See instruction 3c on page 9 for the definition of sponsorship.) Enter "Yes" or "No." ▶..............

4 **ENTITY CODE.** (If not shown, enter the applicable code from page 9 of the instructions.) ▶

5a Name of plan ▶ ....

5b Effective date of plan (mo., day, yr.)

5c Three-digit plan number ▶

All filers must complete 6a through 6d, as applicable.

6a ☐ Welfare benefit plan   6b ☐ Pension benefit plan

(If the correct codes are not preprinted below, enter the applicable codes from page 9 of the instructions in the boxes.)

6c Pension plan features. (If the correct codes are not preprinted below, enter the applicable pension plan feature codes from page 10 of the instructions in the boxes.)

6d ☐ Fringe benefit plan. Attach Schedule F (Form 5500). See instructions.

Under penalties of perjury and other penalties set forth in the instructions, I declare that I have examined this return/report, including accompanying schedules and statements, and to the best of my knowledge and belief, it is true, correct, and complete.

Signature of employer/plan sponsor ▶ .... Date ▶ ....
Type or print name of individual signing for employer/plan sponsor ....
Signature of plan administrator ▶ .... Date ▶ ....
Type or print name of individual signing for plan administrator

For Paperwork Reduction Act Notice, see page 1 of the instructions. Cat. No. 10957K Form **5500-C/R** (1992)

Exhibit 7–3 continued

Form 5500-C/R (1992) **5500-R filers complete this page. 5500-C filers skip this page and complete pages 3 through 6.** Page 2

6e Other plan features: (1) ☐ Master trust (2) ☐ Common/Collective trust (3) ☐ Pooled separate account — Yes | No

7a Total participants: (1) At the beginning of plan year ▶ .... (2) At the end of plan year ▶ ....

b Enter number of participants with account balances at the end of the plan year (defined benefit plans do not complete this item) ▶ ....

c (1) Were any participants in the pension benefit plan separated from service with a deferred vested benefit for which a Schedule SSA (Form 5500) is required to be attached? (See instructions.) . . . . . **7c(1)**

(2) If "Yes," enter the number of separated participants required to be reported ▶

8a Was this plan terminated during this plan year or any prior plan year? If "Yes," enter the year ▶........ **8a**

b Were all the plan assets either distributed to participants or beneficiaries, transferred to another plan, or brought under the control of PBGC? **8b**

c If 8a is "Yes" and the plan is covered by PBGC, is the plan continuing to file PBGC Form 1 and pay premiums until the end of the plan year in which assets are distributed or brought under the control of PBGC? **8c**

9 Is this a plan established or maintained pursuant to one or more collective bargaining agreements? **9**

10 If any benefits are provided by an insurance company, insurance service, or similar organization, enter the number of Schedules A (Form 5500), Insurance Information, that are attached. If none, enter "-0-." ▶

11a (1) Were any plan amendments adopted during this plan year? If "No," complete (2) below and go to item 12a . . . **11a(1)**

(2) Enter the date the most recent amendment was adopted . . . . . ▶ mo. ...... day ..... yr. .....

b If 11a is "Yes," did any amendment result in a retroactive reduction of accrued benefits for any participant? . . . **11b**

c If 11a is "Yes," did any amendment change the information contained in the latest summary plan description or summary description of modifications available at the time of the amendment? **11c**

d If 11c is "Yes," has a summary plan description or summary description of modifications that reflects the plan amendments referred to in 11c been both furnished to participants and filed with the Department of Labor? **11d**

12a If this is a pension benefit plan subject to the minimum funding standards, has the plan experienced a funding deficiency for this plan year? Defined benefit plans must answer this question and attach Schedule B (Form 5500) **12a**

b If 12a is "Yes," have you filed Form 5330 to pay the excise tax? **12b**

13a Total plan assets as of the beginning .... and end .... of the plan year

b Total liabilities as of the beginning .... and end .... of the plan year

c Net assets as of the beginning and end of the plan year

14 For this plan year, enter: a Plan income .... b Expenses .... c Net income (loss) — d Plan contributions .... e Total benefits paid .... (subtract 14b from 14a)

15 The following applies to item 15: (i) you may **NOT** use **N/A** in response to any line item, and (ii) if "Yes" is checked, you must enter a dollar amount in the amount column. — Yes | No | Amount

During this plan year:

a Was this plan covered by a fidelity bond? **15a**

b If 15a is "Yes," enter the name of the surety company ▶ ....

c Was there any loss to the plan, whether or not reimbursed, caused by fraud or dishonesty? . . . **15c**

d Was there any sale, exchange, or lease of any property between the plan and the employer, any fiduciary, any of the five most highly paid employees of the employer, any owner of a 10% or more interest in the employer, or relatives of any such persons? . . . **15d**

e Was there any loan or extension of credit by the plan to the employer, any fiduciary, any of the five most highly paid employees of the employer, any owner of a 10% or more interest in the employer, or relatives of any such persons? **15e**

f Did the plan acquire or hold any employer security or employer real property? **15f**

g Has the plan granted an extension on any delinquent loan owed to the plan? **15g**

h Has the employer owed contributions to the plan which are more than 3 months overdue? . . . **15h**

i Were any loans by the plan or fixed income obligations due the plan classified as uncollectible or in default as of the close of the plan year? **15i**

j Has any plan fiduciary had a financial interest in excess of 10% in any party providing services to the plan or received anything of value from any such party? **15j**

k Did the plan at any time hold 20% or more of its assets in any single security, debt, mortgage, parcel of real estate, or partnership/joint venture interests? **15k**

l Did the plan at any time engage in any transaction or series of related transactions involving 20% or more of the current value of plan assets? **15l**

m Were there any noncash contributions made to the plan the value of which was set without an appraisal by an independent third party? **15m**

n Were there any purchases of nonpublicly traded securities by the plan the value of which was set without an appraisal by an independent third party? **15n**

o Has the plan reduced or failed to provide any benefit when due under the plan because of insufficient assets? . **15o**

16a Is the plan covered under the Pension Benefit Guaranty Corporation termination insurance program? ☐ Yes ☐ No ☐ Not determined

b If 16a is "Yes" or "Not determined," enter the employer identification number and the plan number used to identify it.

Employer identification number ▶ Plan number ▶

Exhibit 7–3 continued

Form 5500-C/R (1992) **5500-C filers complete this page and pages 4 through 6. (See instructions on page 13.)** Page **3**

6e Check all applicable investment arrangements below (see instructions):
(1) ☐ Master trust (2) ☐ 103-12 investment entity
(3) ☐ Common/collective trust (4) ☐ Pooled separate account

....

....

....

....

f Single-employer plans enter the tax year end of the employer in which this plan year ends ▶ Month .... Day .... Year ....

g Is any part of this plan funded by an insurance contract described in Code section 412(i)? . . . . ☐ Yes ☐ No

h If 6g is "Yes," was the part subject to the minimum funding standards for either of the prior two plan years? . . . ☐ Yes ☐ No

7a Total participants: (1) At the beginning of plan year ▶ .... (2) At the end of plan year ▶ ....

b Enter number of participants with account balances at the end of the plan year. (Defined benefits plans do not complete this item.) ▶ ....

c Number of participants that terminated employment during the plan year with accrued benefits that were less than 100% vested ▶ ....

		Yes	No
d (1) Were any participants in the pension benefit plan separated from service with a deferred vested benefit for which a Schedule SSA (Form 5500) is required to be attached?	7d(1)		
(2) If "Yes," enter the number of separated participants required to be reported ▶			
8a Was this plan ever amended since its effective date? If "Yes," complete 8b and, if the amendment was adopted in this plan year, complete 8c through 8e	8a		
b If 8a is "Yes," enter the date the most recent amendment was adopted ▶ Month .... Day .... Year			
c Did any amendment during the current plan year result in the retroactive reduction of accrued benefits for any participant?	8c		
d During this plan year, did any amendment change the information contained in the latest summary plan description or summary description of modifications available at the time of amendment?	8d		
e If 8d is "Yes," has a summary plan description or summary description of modifications that reflects the plan amendments referred to in 8d been both furnished to participants and filed with the Department of Labor?	8e		
9a Was this plan terminated during this plan year or any prior plan year? If "Yes," enter year ▶	9a		
b Were all plan assets either distributed to participants or beneficiaries, transferred to another plan, or brought under the control of PBGC?	9b		
c Was a resolution to terminate this plan adopted during this plan year or any prior plan year?	9c		
d If 9a or 9c is "Yes," have you received a favorable determination letter from the IRS for the termination?	9d		
e If 9d is "No," has a determination letter been requested from the IRS?	9e		
f If 9a or 9c is "Yes," have participants and beneficiaries been notified of the termination or the proposed termination? .	9f		
g If 9a is "Yes" and the plan is covered by PBGC, is the plan continuing to file a PBGC Form 1 and pay premiums until the end of the plan year in which assets are distributed or brought under the control of PBGC?	9g		
h During this plan year, did any trust assets revert to the employer for which the Code section 4980 excise tax is due? .	9h		
i If 9h is "Yes," enter the amount of tax paid with Form 5330 ▶ $			
10a Was this plan merged or consolidated into another plan(s), or were assets or liabilities transferred to another plan(s) since the end of the plan year covered by the last return/report Form 5500 or 5500-C which was filed for this plan (or during this plan year if this is the first return/report)? If "Yes," complete 10b through 10e, and see the instructions for 9a to complete item 9 if the plan was terminated	10a		

If "Yes," identify the other plan(s):

b Name of plan(s) ▶	**c** Employer identification number(s)	**d** Plan number(s)
....	....	....
....	....	....

e If required, has a Form 5310-A been filed? . . . . ☐ Yes ☐ No

11 Enter the plan funding arrangement code from page 14 of the instructions ▶	**12** Enter the plan benefit arrangement code from page 14 of the instructions ▶		Yes	No
13 Is this a plan established or maintained pursuant to one or more collective bargaining agreements?		13		
14 If any benefits are provided by an insurance company, insurance service, or similar organization, enter the number of Schedules A (Form 5500), Insurance Information, that are attached. If none, enter "-0-." ▶				

Exhibit 7–3 continued

Form 5500-C/R (1992) Page 4

Welfare Plans Do Not Complete Items 15 Through 25. Skip To Item 26.

			Yes	No
15a	If this is a defined benefit plan subject to the minimum funding standards for this plan year, is Schedule B (Form 5500) required to be attached? (If this is a defined contribution plan, leave blank.) If "Yes," attach Schedule B (Form 5500).	15a		
b	If this is a defined contribution plan (i.e., money purchase or target benefit), is it subject to the minimum funding standards (if a waiver was granted, see instructions)? (If this is a defined benefit plan, leave blank.) If "Yes," complete (1), (2), and (3) below:	15b		
	(1) Amount of employer contribution required for the plan year under Code section 412 — 15b(1) $			
	(2) Amount of contribution paid by the employer for the plan year — 15b(2) $. Enter date of last payment by employer ▶ Month ..... Day ...... Year			
	(3) If (1) is greater than (2), subtract (2) from (1) and enter the funding deficiency here. Otherwise, enter -0-. (If you have a funding deficiency, file Form 5330.) — 15b(3) $			
16	Has the annual compensation of each participant taken into account under the current plan year been limited to $228,860?	16		
17a	(1) Did the plan distribute any annuity contracts this year? (See instructions.)	17a(1)		
	(2) If (1) is "Yes," did these contracts contain a requirement that the spouse consent before any distributions under the contract are made in a form other than a qualified joint and survivor annuity?	17a(2)		
b	Did the plan make distributions to participants or beneficiaries in a form other than a qualified joint and survivor annuity (a life annuity if a single person) or a qualified preretirement survivor annuity (exclude deferred annuity contracts)?	17b		
c	Did the plan make distributions or loans to married participants and beneficiaries without the required consent of the participant's spouse?	17c		
d	Upon plan amendment or termination, do the accrued benefits of every participant include the subsidized benefits that the participant may become entitled to receive subsequent to the plan amendment or termination?	17d		
18	Were distributions, if any, made in accordance with the requirements of Code sections 411(a)(11) and 417(e)? (See instructions.)	18		
19	Have any contributions been made or benefits accrued in excess of the Code section 415 limits, as amended by the Tax Reform Act of 1986?	19		
20	Has the plan made the required distributions in 1992 under Code section 401(a)(9)? (See instructions.)	20		
21	Check if you are applying either of the following in completing items 21a through 21o (see instructions): (i) ☐ Reasonable, good faith interpretation of the nondiscrimination provisions (ii) ☐ Substantiation guidelines. If you checked 21(ii), enter the first day of the plan year for which data is being submitted ▶ mo. ... day .. yr. ...			
a	Does the employer apply the separate line of business rules of Code section 414(r) when testing this plan for the coverage and discrimination tests requirements of Code sections 410(b) and 401(a)(4)?	21a		
b	If 21a is "Yes," enter the total number of separate lines of business claimed by the employer ▶ .... If more than one separate line of business, see instructions for additional information to attach.			
c	Does the employer apply the mandatory disaggregation rules under Income Tax Regulations section 1.410(b)–7(c)? If "Yes," see instructions for additional information to attach	21c		
d	In testing whether this plan satisfies the coverage and discrimination tests of Code sections 410(b) and 401(a), does the employer aggregate plans?	21d		
e	Does the employer restructure the plan into component plans to satisfy the coverage and discrimination tests of Code sections 410(b) and 401(a)(4)?	21e		
f	If you meet either one of the following exceptions, check the applicable box to tell us which exception you meet and do NOT complete the rest of question 21: (1) ☐ No highly compensated employee benefited under the plan at any time during the plan year; (2) ☐ This is a collectively bargained plan that benefits only collectively bargained employees, no more than 2% of whom are professional employees.			
g	Did any leased employee perform services for the employer at any time during the plan year?	21g		
			Number	
h	Enter the total number of employees of the employer. Employer includes entities aggregated with the employer under Code section 414(b), (c), or (m). Include leased employees and self-employed individuals	21h		
i	Enter the total number of employees excludable under the plan because of: *(1)* failure to meet requirements for minimum age and years of service; *(2)* collectively bargained employees; *(3)* nonresident aliens who receive no earned income from U. S. sources; and *(4)* minimum hours of service/last day rule?	21i		

Exhibit 7–3 continued

Form 5500-C/R (1992) Page **5**

			Number
j	Enter the number of nonexcludable employees (subtract line 21l from line 21h)	21j	
k	Do 100% of the nonexcludable employees entered on line 21j benefit under the plan? ☐ Yes ☐ No If line 21k is "Yes," do NOT complete lines 21l through 21o.		
l	Enter the number of nonexcludable employees (line 21j) who are highly compensated employees	21l	
m	Enter the number of nonexcludable employees who benefit under the plan	21m	
n	Enter the number of employees entered on line 21m who are highly compensated employees	21n	
o	This plan satisfies the coverage requirements on the basis of (check one): (1) ☐ The average benefits test (2) ☐ The ratio percentage test—enter value ▶		

			Yes	No
22a	Is it or was it ever intended that this plan qualify under Code section 401(a)? If "Yes," complete 22b and 22c	22a		
b	Enter the date of the most recent IRS determination letter. Month .... Year			
c	Is a determination letter request pending with the IRS?	22c		
23a	Does the plan hold any assets that have a fair market value that is not readily determinable on an established market? (If "Yes," answer 23b.)	23a		
b	Were all the assets referred to in 23a valued during the 1992 plan year by an independent third-party appraiser?	23b		
c	If 23b is "No," enter the value of the assets that were not valued by an independent third-party appraiser during the 1992 plan year ▶ 23c			
d	Enter the date the assets in 23c were valued by an independent third-party appraiser. (If more than one date, enter the earliest date.) ▶ .... (If this plan has NO ESOP features, leave 23e blank and go to 24.)			
e	If dividends paid on employer securities held by the ESOP were used to make payments on ESOP loans, enter the amount of the dividends used to make the payments ▶ 23e			
24	Does the employer/sponsor listed in 1a of this form maintain other qualified pension benefit plans? If "Yes," enter the total number of plans, including this plan ▶	24		

25a Is the plan covered under the Pension Benefit Guaranty Corporation termination insurance program? ☐ Yes ☐ No ☐ Not determined

b If 25a is "Yes" or "Not determined," enter the employer identification number and the plan number used to identify it.
Employer identification number ▶ Plan number ▶

			Yes	No	Amount
26	The following applies to item 26: (i) you may NOT use N/A in response to any line item, and (ii) if "Yes" is checked, you must enter a dollar amount in the amount column. **During this plan year:**				
a	Was this plan covered by a fidelity bond?	26a			
b	If 26a is "Yes," enter the name of the surety company ▶				
c	Was there any loss to the plan, whether or not reimbursed, caused by fraud or dishonesty?	26c			
d	Was there any sale, exchange, or lease of any property between the plan and the employer, any fiduciary, any of the five most highly paid employees of the employer, any owner of a 10% or more interest in the employer, or relatives of any such persons?	26d			
e	Was there any loan or extension of credit by the plan to the employer, any fiduciary, any of the five most highly paid employees of the employer, any owner of a 10% or more interest in the employer, or relatives of any such persons?	26e			
f	Did the plan acquire or hold any employer security or employer real property?	26f			
g	Has the plan granted an extension on any delinquent loan owed to the plan?	26g			
h	Has the employer owed contributions to the plan which are more than 3 months overdue?	26h			
i	Were any loans by the plan or fixed income obligations due the plan classified as uncollectible or in default as of the close of the plan year?	26i			
j	Has any plan fiduciary had a financial interest in excess of 10% in any party providing services to the plan or received anything of value from any such party?	26j			
k	Did the plan at any time hold 20% or more of its assets in any single security, debt, mortgage, parcel of real estate, or partnership/joint venture interests?	26k			
l	Did the plan at any time engage in any transaction or series of related transactions involving 20% or more of the current value of plan assets?	26l			
m	Were there any noncash contributions made to the plan whose value was set without an appraisal by an independent third party?	26m			
n	Were there any purchases of nonpublicly traded securities by the plan whose value was set without an appraisal by an independent third party?	26n			
o	Has the plan reduced or failed to provide any benefit when due under the terms of the plan because of insufficient assets?	26o			

Exhibit 7–3 continued

Form 5500-C/R (1992) Page 6

27 Current value of plan assets and liabilities at the beginning and end of the plan year. Combine the value of plan assets held in more than one trust. Allocate the value of the plan's interest in a commingled trust containing the assets of more than one plan on a line-by-line basis unless the trust meets one of the specific exceptions described in the instructions. Do not enter the value of the portion of an insurance contract which guarantees during this plan year to pay a specific dollar benefit at a future date. **Round off amounts to the nearest dollar. Any other amounts are subject to rejection. Plans with no assets at the beginning and end of the plan year enter -0- on line 27f.**

		(a) Beginning of year	(b) End of year
Assets			
a Cash	27a		
b Receivables	27b		
c Investments:			
(1) U.S. Government securities	27c(1)		
(2) Corporate debt and equity instruments	27c(2)		
(3) Real estate and mortgages (other than to participants)	27c(3)		
(4) Loans to participants:			
A Mortgages	(4)A		
B Other	(4)B		
(5) Other	27c(5)		
(6) Total investments (add (1) through (5)) ▶	27c(6)		
d Buildings and other property used in plan operations	27d		
e Other assets	27e		
f Total assets (add a, b, c(6), d, and e) ▶	27f		
Liabilities			
g Payables	27g		
h Acquisition indebtedness	27h		
i Other liabilities	27i		
j Total liabilities (add g through i) ▶	27j		
k Net assets (f minus j) ▶	27k		

28 Plan income, expenses, and changes in net assets for the plan year. Include all income and expenses of the plan including any trust(s) or separately maintained fund(s) and any payments/receipts to/from insurance carriers. **Round off amounts to the nearest dollar. Any other amounts are subject to rejection.**

		(a) Amount	(b) Total
Income			
a Contributions received or receivable in cash from:			
(1) Employer(s) (including contributions on behalf of self-employed individuals)	28a(1)		
(2) Employees	28a(2)		
(3) Others	28a(3)		
(4) Add (1) through (3)	28a(4)		
b Noncash contributions (enter total of a(4) and b in column (b))	28b		
c Earnings from investments (interest, dividends, rents, royalties)	28c		
d Net realized gain (loss) on sale or exchange of assets	28d		
e Other income (specify) ▶	28e		
f Total income (add b through e) ▶	28f		
Expenses			
g Distribution of benefits and payments to provide benefits:			
(1) Directly to participants or their beneficiaries	28g(1)		
(2) Other	28g(2)		
(3) Total distribution of benefits and payments to provide benefits	28g(3)		
h Administrative expenses (salaries, fees, commissions, insurance premiums)	28h		
i Other expenses (specify) ▶	28i		
j Total expenses (add g through i) ▶	28j		
k Net income (loss) (subtract j from f) ▶	28k		

☆ U.S. GOVERNMENT PRINTING OFFICE: 1993 315-063

Exhibit 7–3 continued

SCHEDULE SSA (Form 5500)

Department of the Treasury
Internal Revenue Service

Annual Registration Statement Identifying Separated Participants With Deferred Vested Benefits

Under Section 6057(a) of the Internal Revenue Code

▶ File as an attachment to Form 5500 or 5500-C/R.

▶ For Paperwork Reduction Act Notice, see page 1 of the instructions for Form 5500 or 5500-C/R.

OMB No. 1210-0016

1992

This Form is NOT Open to Public Inspection

For the calendar year 1992 or fiscal plan year beginning , 1992, and ending , 19

▶ **This schedule must be filed for each plan year in which one or more participants with deferred vested benefit rights separated from the service covered by the plan. See instructions on when to report a separated employee.**

▶ **Type or print in ink all entries on this schedule. File the originals.**

▶ **All attachments to this schedule should have entries only on the front of the page.**

1a Name of sponsor (employer if for a single employer plan)

1b Sponsor's employer identification number

Number, street, and room or suite no. (If a P.O. box, see the instructions for 1a.)

1c Is this a plan to which more than one employer contributes? . . ☐ **Yes** ☐ **No**

City or town, state, and ZIP code

2a Name of plan administrator (if other than sponsor)

2b Administrator's employer identification no.

Number, street, and room or suite no. (If a P.O. box, see the instructions for 1a.)

City or town, state, and ZIP code

3a Name of plan

3b Plan number. ▶

4 Have you notified each separated participant of his or her deferred benefit? . . . . ▶ ☐ **Yes** ☐ **No**

5 Separated participants with deferred vested benefits (if additional space is required, see instruction, "What To File"):

(a) Social security number	(b) Name of participant	Enter code for nature and form of benefit		Amount of vested benefit			(h) Plan year in which participant separated
		(c) Type of annuity	(d) Payment frequency	(e) Defined benefit plan—periodic payment	Defined contribution plan: (f) Units or shares	Defined contribution plan: (g) Total value of account	

The Following Information Is Optional (See Specific Instruction 6.)

6 Use this item to report: (i) separated participants with deferred vested benefits who were previously reported on Schedule SSA (Form 5500) and who have received part or all of their vested benefits or who have forfeited their benefits during the plan year for which this schedule is being filed, and (ii) to delete participants erroneously reported on a prior Schedule SSA (Form 5500).

Note: *Participants listed in this item, because they have received part of their vested benefits, must also be reported in item 5 above listing their remaining vested benefits.*

(a) Social security number	(b) Name of participant	Enter code for nature and form of benefit		Amount of vested benefit			(h) Plan year in which participant separated
		(c) Type of annuity	(d) Payment frequency	(e) Defined benefit plan—periodic payment	Defined contribution plan: (f) Units or shares	Defined contribution plan: (g) Total value of account	

Under penalties of perjury, I declare that I have examined this report, and to the best of my knowledge and belief, it is true, correct, and complete.

Signature of plan administrator ▶ **Date ▶**

Cat. No. 13506T **Schedule SSA (Form 5500) (1992)**

Exhibit 7–3 continued

SCHEDULE P (Form 5500)
Department of the Treasury
Internal Revenue Service

Annual Return of Fiduciary of Employee Benefit Trust

▶ File as an attachment to Form 5500, 5500-C/R, or 5500EZ.
▶ For the Paperwork Reduction Notice, see page 1 of the Form 5500 instructions.

OMB No. 1210-0016

1992

For trust calendar year 1992 or fiscal year beginning , 1992, and ending , 19

Please type or print

1a Name of trustee or custodian

b Number, street, and room or suite no. (If a P.O. box, see the instructions for Form 5500, 5500-C/R, or 5500EZ.)

c City or town, state, and ZIP code

2a Name of trust

b Trust's employer identification number

3 Name of plan if different from name of trust

4 Have you furnished the participating employee benefit plan(s) with the trust financial information required to be reported by the plan(s)? . . . . ☐ Yes ☐ No

5 Enter the plan sponsor's employer identification number as shown on Form 5500, 5500-C/R, or 5500EZ . . . . ▶

Under penalties of perjury, I declare that I have examined this schedule, and to the best of my knowledge and belief it is true, correct, and complete.

Signature of fiduciary ▶ Date ▶

Instructions

(Section references are to the Internal Revenue Code.)

Purpose of Form

You may use this schedule to satisfy the requirements under section 6033(a) for an annual information return from every section 401(a) organization exempt from tax under section 501(a).

Filing this form will start the running of the statute of limitations under section 6501(a) for any trust described in section 401(a), which is exempt from tax under section 501(a).

Who May File

1. Every trustee of a trust created as part of an employee benefit plan as described in section 401(a).

2. Every custodian of a custodial account described in section 401(f).

How To File

File Schedule P (Form 5500) for the trust year ending with or within any participating plan's plan year. Attach it to the Form 5500, 5500-C/R, or 5500EZ filed by the plan for that plan year. A separately filed Schedule P (Form 5500) will not be accepted.

If the trust or custodial account is used by more than one plan, file one Schedule P (Form 5500). If a plan uses more than one trust or custodial account for its funds, file one Schedule P (Form 5500) for each trust or custodial account.

Signature

The fiduciary (trustee or custodian) must sign this schedule. If there is more than one fiduciary, the fiduciary authorized by the others may sign.

Other Returns and Forms That May Be Required

- **Form 990-T.**—For trusts described in section 401(a), a tax is imposed on income derived from business that is unrelated to the purpose for which the trust received a tax exemption. Report this income and tax on **Form 990-T,** Exempt Organization Business Income Tax Return. (See sections 511 through 514 and the related regulations.)
- **Form 1099-R.**—If you made payments or distributions to individual beneficiaries of a plan, report those payments on Form 1099-R. (See sections 6041 and 6047 and the related regulations.)
- **Forms 941 or 941E.**—If you made payments or distributions to individual beneficiaries of a plan, you are required to withhold income tax from those payments unless the payee elects not to have the tax withheld. Report any withholding tax on Form 941 or 941E. (See Form 941 or 941E, and **Circular E,** Employer's Tax Guide (Pub. 15), for more information.

Cat. No. 13504X

Schedule P (Form 5500) 1992

INSERT

TAB

◆ Part III ◆

Personal Financial Planning

◆ Chapter 8 ◆

The Short Course on Personal Finances

LESSON 8–1: WHAT EXACTLY ARE WE TRYING TO ACCOMPLISH?

I have a confession. When I was about 30 years old and many of my clients were 50 or 60, I would prepare elaborate personal financial plans for them. These included income statements, balance sheets, budgets, a list of financial goals, and so on. The reports looked great.

As I grew older, I realized that those elaborate plans were largely unnecessary. Now, before I sit down with a physician and spouse to discuss personal finances, I have them complete a questionnaire. The questionnaire gathers the usual financial information, but I have added a page that asks, "What is it that you really want?"

I ask clients to grade, on a scale of 1 to 10, a series of financial planning objectives. The grade depends on how important each objective is to them. Here are some examples:

- Retire early.
- Provide for the college education for children.
- Pay off home mortgage.
- Maintain current standard of living.

- Retire at current standard of living.
- Contribute to charity.
- Budget expenses better.
- Take care of family in the event of death or disability.
- Travel more.
- Accumulate wealth for heirs.
- Minimize estate taxes.
- Minimize income taxes.
- Save money.
- Reduce debts.

I have compiled the results of dozens of these questionnaires. Based on what my wise clients have told me, these are the financial objectives that most physicians desire:

- Buy a nice home for family.
- Provide for children's education.
- Provide for retirement.
- Try to save about 10% of income each year.
- Avoid unwise investments.
- Stay out of debt.
- Provide for family in the event of death or disability.
- Give some time and money back to the community.
- Whatever money is left over, spend and enjoy. Life passes so quickly.

The rest of this chapter will discuss how to attain these nine goals and avoid pitfalls along the way.

LESSON 8–2: THE PHYSICIAN'S BIGGEST PERSONAL FINANCIAL MISTAKE

Louisiana is a peculiar place. Among its peculiarities is a tree that grows tall and full at its top yet has a small, shallow root system. Every time I ask what kind of tree this is, people tell me, "That's an old trash tree. It ain't good for nothing."

Louisiana is also known for storms and hurricanes. As you can imagine, these top-heavy trash trees don't do well in strong winds. It is common after a storm to see several of these trees collapsed under the weight of their own imprudent growth. And so it is with some of us.

The single biggest mistake physicians make in the management of their finances is debt, debt, debt.

There is an irony here. The catastrophe that physicians fear most is the infamous malpractice award that exceeds the limits of their insurance coverage and wipes them out personally.

Almost every physician mentions this fear, yet I have never met a physician who lost one cent of his or her personal assets to a malpractice award. I have, however, met several physicians who have lost significant portions of their personal wealth, and been forced into bankruptcy, because of that four-letter word: debt. Today, it is far too easy to borrow too much money. The consequence of easy credit is the years of additional work necessary to pay off that debt. The newest twist on cute debt is the second mortgage. It is now considered wise to buy a car or go on a vacation with money borrowed and secured by a second mortgage on the house. What inevitably happens is that the car is traded, the vacation ends, and all that remains, for years and years, is debt.

My best advice:

- Long-term debts (those that will be paid back over a period longer than one year) must always be associated with an asset such as a house or car that will be useful at least as long as the debt. (Tip: When mortgaging your house, try to obtain a 15-year mortgage instead of the traditional 30-year mortgage. The increase in your monthly payment is modest, and the interest savings is phenomenal.)
- Assets that are purchased with long-term debt must have a value that is at least equal to the remaining balance of the debt. In other words, you should be able to sell your car or your house and completely pay off the debt associated with it.
- Don't borrow funds for consumables such as vacations, watches, or furs. Lifestyle loans are treacherous because the original purchase is soon a memory or out of style and the debt seems to hang on forever.
- Pay off your credit card balances every month. If this is difficult, I recommend the American Express card, which requires that the monthly balance be paid in full. As for other cards and their nondeductible 18% and higher interest rates, burn 'em.

- I would like to say never, but instead I will say be extremely careful about borrowing money to make an investment. Most of the real financial tragedies that I have seen are the result of borrowing money or signing notes for that can't-miss real estate investment, tugboat, barge, or oil and gas well.
- The total amount of all your payments for long- and short- term debts should never exceed 35% of your gross pay.

Debt really isn't as American as apple pie. If you can entirely avoid being in debt, do so. If, like most of us, you find that you need to assume some debt, do so sparingly and with a keen eye as to the present and future value of the asset you are about to purchase.

Just as it is true that cash will always be king, it is also true that the borrower will always be a slave to the lender. When it comes to debt, your goal should be to set yourself free from it as soon as possible.

LESSON 8–3: THE TEN COMMANDMENTS OF INVESTING

Ah, the perils of investing. It used to be so simple. Banks offered passbook savings accounts and certificates of deposit. Stockbrokers sold stocks and bonds. That was it. Now, everyone sells everything, and the products they sell are as varied as the promises they make.

Times have indeed become complex when you can borrow money at a lower interest rate from your stockbroker than from your banker and buy stock cheaper from your banker than your broker.

Not complicated enough? Walk into today's department stores. Amidst the clothes and the refrigerators, you will find an insurance agent, a real estate agent, and a stockbroker all waiting to be of service. What this all adds up to is more businesses than ever before saying, "Give me your money." Where do you turn?

It would take a dozen books to explain every investment product available in the marketplace today. The purpose of this lesson is to provide you with 10 basic rules to apply to each and every investment decision you face. This is the 10-step "smell test":

1. Now, as in the past, and forevermore: If it sounds too good to be true, it is!
2. Never buy any investment that you do not thoroughly understand, and never buy an investment sold unsolicited over the telephone. Do not succumb to high-pressure sales tactics. Sometimes the most prudent investment words you can speak are, "No, I am not interested."
3. Build your investment portfolio slowly and consistently. You must discipline yourself to save and invest money on a regular basis. If you put off saving and investing until a better time, when you have more cash, that time will never come.
4. If you do not have the temperament for a particular investment, don't buy it. For example, if you have invested in a stock and find that the day-to-day fluctuations in the price of that stock are causing heart palpitations, you probably are not suited for investing in the stock market. If you have found this out after buying a particular investment, it is still probably better to sell the stock and learn from the experience.
5. Be conservative. Don't fall for wild stories about doubling and tripling your money in a short period of time. Home run stories about people who bought investments that shot up in value instantly are great to hear but, in reality, seldom exist. Stupidity stories are seldom heard but exist in abundance. Too many people invest poorly because someone told them what they wanted to hear. Don't get greedy.
6. The real winners are the day-in, day-out consistent investments. Stick with them. Remember, your investment portfolio needs to be built on solid rock. Therefore, it should be made up of prudent, well-diversified investments that you fully understand.

7. Monitor your investment portfolio, and never be afraid to take gains or losses. There is an old stock market adage: "Bulls make money, bears make money, and pigs get slaughtered."
8. All investments require thorough knowledge on your part. Never let any expert invest your money without your supervision. Advisors have an important role in your finances: They advise. Only you can make final decisions.
9. Don't invest money with someone just because he or she shares your race, religion, occupation, or club membership.
10. Finally, use your common sense. Common sense, a precious commodity, is often sidetracked by enthusiasm. Always ask yourself whether the investment makes sense. Don't ask whether the person selling the investment makes sense because pitches are always logical and polished. If the investment doesn't make sense to you, pass.

If this sounds like plain vanilla advice, it is. This is exactly how it is meant to sound. All too often, common sense is the best advice I have to offer a zealous client. I have heard far too many stories that started with great promises and ended up as tales of tragic losses.

Unfortunately, people work so hard for their money and part with it far too hastily. Lines such as *great investment, no-risk, unbelievable rate of return, can't fail,* and *hurry up or you'll miss out* should be met with skepticism, not open arms. Financial markets are efficient. This means that supply and demand tend to keep them constant. Interest rates and other investments offered in New York will usually be similar to those offered in Tucson, Arizona or Butte, Montana. If someone promises you a deal significantly better than the current market rate, beware, even if that someone is a large national firm or a supposed expert.

LESSON 8–4: RISKY BUSINESS

> The race is not to the swift or the battle to the strong nor does food come to the wise or wealth to the brilliant or favor to the learned; but time and chance happen to them all. Moreover, no man knows when his hour will come.
>
> Ecclesiastes 9:11–12*

Insurance. No topic causes more eyes to roll or telephone messages to go unanswered. So I'll be brief. There are two kinds of insurance that you will be urged to purchase throughout your career: life insurance and disability insurance. Chances are that you will need both coverages. This lesson will explain the basics of each.

Life Insurance

Why they call it life insurance I will never know. Life insurance neither insures that you will live nor pays you for doing so. In reality, it is death insurance. I suppose that the life insurance industry would find it considerably more difficult to peddle their wares if they were appropriately named.

Do you need life insurance? To answer this question, you must first determine whether you have a true need for life insurance. In short, if you died today, would anyone be dependent on your continued support?

All insurance is really a form of *risk management*. For instance, there is a statistically small chance that some event could cause a financial disaster. Your house could burn down, or a car accident or a serious illness could cause death or disability. These are all examples of risks that are managed through insurance. Life insurance should be part of your risk management portfolio, not your investment portfolio. Life insurance is designed to provide funds for those who would suffer financially from your premature death. If no one depends on you financially, then despite the barrage of arguments offered by insurance agents you do not need life insurance.

Marriage may not automatically create a life insurance need. If your family consists of just you and your spouse and both of you have high-paying jobs, there still may not be a need for life insurance. The true need for insurance on your life usually begins with the arrival of children.

How much life insurance do you need? Insurance companies usually offer snappy little formulas for calculating insurance needs based on your salary. Most of these formulas are of questionable worth, serving only to prod you into buying more insurance than you need.

---

*Taken from the HOLY BIBLE, NEW INTERNATIONAL VERSION copyright 1973, 1978 by the International Bible Society, used by permission of Zondervan Bible Publishers.

The most accurate method of determining the amount of life insurance you need is the needs analysis worksheet (Exhibit 8–1).

Once you have calculated how much life insurance you need, you will face the even more difficult question of which type of insurance to buy. Three basic options are available: term life insurance, whole life insurance, and universal life insurance.

What type of insurance is best? Term life insurance is basic life insurance protection for a specific period of time. With term insurance, you do not build up cash surrender value. Term insurance provides a death benefit for a specified period of time. Policies are usually issued in one-year increments. Some term insurance is guaranteed renewable. This means that, as long as you pay the annual premium, coverage is guaranteed in future years, usually up to age 65.

Exhibit 8–1 Current Insurance Needs Analysis Worksheet

1. Your annual income		$________
2. If married, your spouse's annual income..................	+	$________
TOTAL FAMILY INCOME		$________
3. What percentage of this total is needed to maintain your family's standard of living (We recommend 75%)	×	________%
SUBTOTAL...		________
4. Subtract spouse's portion of the income if he/she plans to continue working after you die	−	________
SUBTOTAL...		________
5. Subtract annual income from other sources	−	________
SUBTOTAL...		________
6. Divide by a reasonable interest rate you would likely earn by investing a lump sum of cash. For example, if 7% sounds reasonable, divide by .07; if 9% sounds reasonable, divide by .09....	÷	________
SUBTOTAL...		________
7. Add estate settlement costs (taxes, probate and funeral expenses). Figure 4 to 6% of your total gross estate	+	________
8. Add any outstanding mortgage balances	+	________
9. Add education funds	+	________
10. Add unique annual personal expenses (for instance, financial obligations for a disabled parent or a handicapped child)	+	________
SUBTOTAL...		________
11. Subtract existing insurance policies, and other liquid assets such as CDs, stocks, bank account balances, etc.	−	________
APPROXIMATE LIFE INSURANCE NEEDS AT PRESENT	=	________

Source: Reprinted from *Aide Magazine,* August 1991, USAA, San Antonio, Texas, © 1991.

You can purchase term insurance in one of two basic forms. If you wish the face value (death benefit) of the policy to remain the same each year, you would buy level term insurance. Because your chances of dying increase each year, the premiums for level term insurance increase accordingly each year. If you prefer that your annual premium remain constant, then you will need to purchase decreasing term insurance, which has a constant annual premium and a death benefit that decreases annually.

Usually, after age 65 the cost of term insurance is prohibitive, and policies are allowed to expire. By that time, however, you should have your children educated and out of the house, your financial plan in order, and adequate retirement funds saved. Your life insurance needs should be significantly reduced.

Some term policies will allow you to convert them into whole life policies at specific intervals during the life of the policy. Term insurance is easy to shop for because it is pure insurance. One policy is relatively easy to compare with another. Beware, however, because premiums for term insurance vary considerably. Your best bet is to shop around to find a sound insurance company licensed to sell insurance in your state that offers the best premium.

Term insurance usually best meets the needs of young physicians on limited salaries. It provides high death benefit coverage at low rates. In one's young family years, death benefit coverage is the most important goal of life insurance. Despite arguments to the contrary, the best way to achieve this goal on a limited budget is with term insurance.

Whole life insurance is a permanent insurance plan that offers both a death benefit and a cash surrender value. It is the most widely sold life insurance. It pays out the highest commissions to insurance agents and can be pushed hard by them.

In a typical whole life policy, you pay a level premium for a period of several years in exchange for a fixed death benefit. Your premium is used by the insurance company to accomplish a variety of tasks. Part of the premium goes to pay the agent's commission; part is used, in essence, to buy a term insurance contract for you; part goes to cover administrative costs; and part is invested on your behalf. It is this forced savings portion, or cash surrender value, that causes so much controversy. The cash surrender value of a policy accumulates on a tax-deferred basis and is returned to you along with dividends if you cash in the policy. The problem is this: Historically, insurance companies have paid low dividend rates, which means that insurance policies were not particularly good investments.

This is beginning to change. Dividend payouts have been increased, mortality tables improved, and policy administrative costs cut to make life insurance more competitive as an investment. At one time, I believed in the general philosophy of buying term insurance and investing the difference yourself. After several years of watching people's spending habits, however, I know that in reality most people buy term insurance and spend the rest on life style.

In certain instances, forced savings is not so bad. For instance, let's say that you have a newborn child. Usually, each new child will increase the amount of life insurance you need and will prompt you to increase the amount set aside for future educational expenses. A good life insurance policy may be a way to accomplish both goals. The policy itself will obviously provide the additional death benefit coverage. The cash surrender value can be structured so that, over an 18-year period, enough funds accumulate to pay for your child's education.

Universal or variable life insurance is similar to whole life insurance in that it offers both a death benefit and cash surrender value. These policies also offer flexibility. You may change the premium payment or the death benefit as needed. This hybrid form of insurance is the insurance industry's answer to a problem it created. Individual policyholders were fed up with the low rates of return on whole life policies and began to demand policies with more competitive yields. Hence the birth of universal and variable life insurance.

Universal and variable life insurance is similar to whole life in most respects except that the forced savings portion of your premium is invested more aggressively, thereby (it is hoped) offering a higher yield.

What is the true cost of a life insurance policy? Cost, in its most basic form, is the difference between what you pay and what you get back from the insurance company. The best way to compare policies is through the use of cost indexes. Cost indexes use several factors, such as premiums paid, cash values, and dividends, to provide you with information that you can use to compare policies.

There are two basic cost indexes: the life insurance surrender cost index, and the life insurance net payment cost index. These indexes are available for all life insurance policies, although you may have to ask your life insurance agent specifically for this information. Generally, the policy with the smaller index number is a better buy than a comparable policy with a larger index number.

How safe is your life insurance company? It is more important than ever to be aware of the financial stability of the company writing your life insurance policies. Here are telephone numbers of companies that rate life insurance companies:

- A.M. Best: 900-420-0400
- Duff & Phelps: 312-368-3175
- Moody's: 212-553-0300
- Standard & Poor's: 212-208-1527
- Weiss Research: 800-289-9222

Disability Insurance

Disability insurance, or income replacement insurance, provides income to you and your family if you become disabled. Statistically, your chances of being disabled are three times greater than your chances of dying prematurely. It is important that you manage the risk of disability through the purchase of a good individual (not group) disability insurance contract.

When buying disability insurance, you should consider the following factors:

- *Definition of disability:* Initially, most policies consider you disabled if you are unable to carry on your specific occupation. For physicians, this would include inability to continue working in their specialty. After a year or two of your being disabled, the policy definition of disability may change. To collect benefits, you would have to be unable to perform any kind of work for which you have experience. This is unacceptable. Good policies will not amend the definition of disability.
- *Waiting period:* Disability policies will pay benefits after an initial waiting period of 30 to 180 days. The longer the waiting period you choose, the less expensive the policy premium. Typically a 90-day waiting period is reasonable for physicians. (Note: This is why experts typically recommend that you have at least three months of salary safely invested as an emergency fund.)
- *Duration of benefits:* Benefit payments can range from five years to life depending on the policy. Life policies are the only ones that I would consider.
- *Other questions to be considered:*
    1. Are guaranteed monthly benefit increases offered at periodic intervals during the life of the policy?
    2. What inflation benefit adjustment options are offered?
    3. What happens if you return to work on a less than full-time basis?
    4. Can the policy be canceled?
    5. Are there any standard exclusions, such as pregnancy?
    6. Is total disability required to receive a benefit?
    7. How are benefits calculated?
    8. How difficult is it to file claims, and where are they processed?
    9. Is vocational rehabilitation offered?
    10. Are premiums waived during the period of disability?

Individually written disability insurance policies are usually expensive, but they are the best policies for physicians. Group policies, although inexpensive, have poor coverages. If you are ever truly disabled, you will be thankful that your policy was written by a good company. There are a handful of companies that write fine individual disability insurance contracts: Provident, The Guardian, Paul Revere, and Northwestern Mutual. The best way to contact these companies is through the local service office in your community. The phone number should be listed in the Yellow Pages.

LESSON 8–5: THE HIGH COST OF HIGHER EDUCATION

It is common for a middle-aged couple to come into my office with stunned looks on their faces. When they finally muster up the strength for words, I hear, "I have two children in college and a third who will be entering in the fall." They pause, give me the "as if that's not bad enough" look, and then add, "The middle child wants a doctorate in fine arts." Finally, they murmur, "What can we do?"

During the 1980s the cost of college tuition, room, and board grew at twice the rate of inflation. In 1993, this translates into an average annual cost of more than $7,000 for state schools and more than $15,000 for private schools. There is no end in sight to these soaring costs. Predictions call for continued increases by approximately 7% a year for the next 20 years. Not a pretty picture.

If you wait until your children are teenagers to begin to fund their higher education, there is little you can do. Often, you will be faced with the unpleasant choice of having to borrow money, place a second mortgage on your home, or dip into funds intended for retirement.

My best advice is as soon as your hear "It's a boy" or "It's a girl," start to save for the child's education. The miracle of compounding is once again the reason for this advice.

How much do you need to save? Exhibit 8–2 consists of an excellent worksheet and tables that you can use to project future education costs. By completing these forms, you will be able to determine how much you will need to save for each child's education and how much per month it will cost.

In whose name should the funds be accumulated? There are three basic methods available to you for accumulating an education fund:

1. *The Uniform Gift to Minors Act (UGMA):* One of the most popular ways to shift income is to open an account under the UGMA. UGMA is recognized in all 50 states and allows you to open an account in your child's name and Social Security number in any bank, homestead, mutual fund, or financial institution. A custodian, usually a parent, is responsible for the account until the child is no longer a minor. You can contribute up to $10,000 per parent per child into these accounts without any gift tax consequences. The income earned in the account is taxed as follows: There is no federal tax on the first $500 of income, a 15% federal tax is applied to the next $500 of income, and all income over $1,000 is taxed at the parents' rate until the child reaches age 14. The major disadvantage of UGMA accounts is that, once the child reaches the age of majority, he or she can legally take the money and spend it on anything.
2. *Educational Trust:* Trust laws vary from state to state, so you will need to discuss specifics with an attorney who specializes in trusts. In general, an educational trust allows for control of the funds even when the child reaches the age of majority. In most instances,

Exhibit 8–2 Worksheet To Compute Future Education Costs

How Much Do You Need To Save?

The calculations on this worksheet are based on the assumption that college costs will rise 7% yearly, a reasonable assumption according to financial planning experts. Fill out the form below using Table A and Table B to assist you in determining your monthly savings amount.

	Your Estimate	Sample Estimate
1. Years to college: You may give yourself more time by using your child's senior college year as your target date.	________	16
2. Current annual cost of tuition, fees, room and board:*	________	$6,546
3. College cost inflation: See Table A to find the inflation factor to use, given your time horizon.	________	2.95
4. Future annual college cost: Multiply #2 by #3.	________	$19,311
5. Future total college cost: Multiply #4 by number of years you expect child will attend college.	________	$77,243
6. After-Tax Rate of Return Factor: See Table B to find the appropriate return factor. Look under your anticipated rate of return and opposite the years remaining to college.	________	25.67
7. Annual savings amount required: Divide #5 by #6.	________	$3,009
8. Monthly savings amount required: Divide #7 by 12.	________	$251

*Two references available through high school guidance counselors provide good average cost figures. They are the College Board's College Cost Book and the ACT's College Planning/Search Book. For 1990–91, the average annual cost of tuition, room and board at a public school was $6,546 and at a private school, $14,570.

Exhibit 8–2 continued

Table A

Years To College	Inflation Factor	Years To College	Inflation Factor
1	1.07	12	2.25
2	1.15	13	2.41
3	1.23	14	2.58
4	1.31	15	2.76
5	1.40	16	2.95
6	1.50	17	3.16
7	1.61	18	3.38
8	1.72	19	3.62
9	1.84	20	3.87
10	1.97	21	4.14
11	2.10		

Table B
Rate of Return Factor

Years To College	3%	4%	5%	6%	7%	8%	9%
1	1.00	1.00	1.00	1.00	1.00	1.00	1.00
2	2.03	2.04	2.05	2.06	2.07	2.08	2.09
3	3.09	3.12	3.15	3.18	3.22	3.25	3.28
4	4.19	4.25	4.31	4.38	4.44	4.51	4.57
5	5.31	5.42	5.53	5.64	5.75	5.87	5.99
6	6.47	6.63	6.80	6.98	7.15	7.34	7.52
7	7.66	7.90	8.14	8.39	8.65	8.92	9.20
8	8.89	9.21	9.55	9.90	10.26	10.64	11.03
9	10.16	10.58	11.03	11.49	11.98	12.49	13.02
10	11.46	12.01	12.58	13.18	13.82	14.49	15.19
11	12.81	13.49	14.21	14.97	15.78	16.65	17.56
12	14.19	15.03	15.92	16.87	17.89	18.98	20.14
13	15.62	16.63	17.71	18.88	20.14	21.50	22.95
14	17.09	18.29	19.60	21.05	22.55	24.22	26.02
15	18.60	20.02	21.58	23.28	25.13	27.15	29.36
16	20.16	21.83	23.66	25.67	27.89	30.32	33.00
17	21.76	23.70	25.84	28.21	30.84	33.75	36.97
18	23.41	25.65	28.13	30.91	34.00	37.45	41.30
19	25.12	27.67	30.54	33.76	37.38	41.45	46.02
20	26.87	29.78	33.07	36.79	41.00	45.76	51.16
21	28.68	31.97	35.72	39.99	44.87	50.42	56.76

Note: This information is copied with permission of The USAA Foundation. Any other usage is expressly prohibited without permission of The USAA Foundation.

an independent trustee must be appointed to administer the trust. All gifts to the trust are irrevocable. Educational trusts are probably most appropriate if you intend to accumulate large sums of money for your heirs.

3. *Educational fund in the parents' name:* This method affords you the most control because the assets in the fund stay in your name. In my opinion, the taxes saved by using a UGMA account or a trust are not enough to risk losing control of the funds. My advice is to establish an educational fund in your name and Social Security number and to fund it monthly or quarterly.

How should I invest the fund? Like your retirement funds, these educational funds should be viewed as long-term, conservative investments. Your best bets are a diversified portfolio of highly rated, no-load stock and bond mutual funds.

There are many excellent publications, such as *Money*, *Kiplinger's*, and *Forbes* that can guide you in selecting appropriate investments for your children's education fund.

LESSON 8–6: OUT OF RESIDENCY AND INTO THE FIRE

It is finally over and just beginning. You have completed your residency and are about to go out into the real world to seek gainful employment. After all your years of technical training, you are about to find out that you are substantially unprepared for one of the major decisions of your life: Where and for whom are you going to work?

On the one hand, you will have many more options available to you than your peers had just 10 years ago. Health maintenance organizations, preferred provider organizations, hospitals, insurance companies, and other types of managed care providers are now hiring more and more physicians directly out of their residencies. Also, of course, single-specialty and multi-specialty groups are vigorously competing for the best and the brightest. On the other hand, because of all these options, selecting the practice arrangement that is best for you is more complicated than ever.

The purpose of this lesson is to aid you in joining your first group and to provide some useful guidelines if you are already in practice and considering changing employment. Money should not be the primary factor in choosing a job. It is likely that you will practice with one group for your entire career, so it is important to give strong consideration to the following questions:

- In what area of the country do I want to practice?
- What type of group am I most comfortable joining?
- What should I expect in an employment contract?

Where Should I Practice?

Where you should practice medicine is obviously a personal decision that will be based primarily on your preferences and personal life style. The good news is that, depending on your specialty, you should have a wide variety of job opportunities available to you throughout the country.

What is important is to choose a locality that suits your life style, a community that you feel comfortable becoming a part of. Check the demographics in the area that you are considering. Is the population growing or shrinking? Is industry moving into or out of the area? What is the most likely scenario for economic growth in the area for the next 10 years? How many other physicians with your specialty already have practices in the area?

You can get a lot of useful information about an area from the local hospital and chamber of commerce. Hospitals and chambers of commerce want you to move into the area, however, so they will usually paint a rosy picture. Carefully interpret and confirm their information. If you are being recruited by a group, the group should also provide you with data that tell you all about the area and the group itself. It is also a good idea to speak to several area physicians who could become referral sources and to get their input on the needs of the community and the opportunities available.

Which Group Is Best for Me?

Once you have determined the area of the country in which you want to practice, the next step is to evaluate the groups recruiting you and the offers they are making. Bear this in mind: Being in a medical group is very similar to being married.

Choose your potential partners carefully because you may be spending the better part of the rest of your life with them. Again, your initial compensation should not be the major consideration in selecting a group. Your major consideration should be, in a word, integrity.

When you are being interviewed, pay close attention to the people in the group. When they describe the practice, is the emphasis on patient care or on productivity? If a group appears to view patients as walking dollar signs, it may very well see you as just another billing unit. How do the physicians treat each other and their staff? These are good indicators of how they will ultimately treat you after the honeymoon is over.

Choosing life-long partners is an extremely important decision. Do everything you can to ensure that the group you are joining places a premium on integrity, teamwork, and quality of patient care.

Among the groups that I have worked with and respect, I have seen many of the following traits:

- Every physician has a say in policymaking. Of course, experienced senior physicians lead the group, but they confer with and listen to all the physicians when making important decisions.
- There is no "mine" versus "yours" attitude. There is a clear understanding that teamwork and compromise make a group stronger.
- There is mutual respect and flexibility that allow physicians to work comfortably with each others' idiosyncrasies. Tough problems and conflicts also are resolved within this framework of "we are partners and need to do what is best for the practice."
- Physicians have lives outside of the practice.

A job interview is a two-way street. Just as the group is trying to determine whether you are the right person to join it, you should be trying to determine whether this is the right group for you. Keep asking yourself throughout the process, "Are these people with whom I can happily spend the rest of my life?"

What Should I Expect in My Contract?

Once you have decided on an area of the country and have found a group to join, the final step is to negotiate your employment contract. I recommend that you get professional help from a lawyer and CPA who are familiar with physician employment contracts. The following is a list of points that are generally addressed in physician employment contracts:

- *Term:* Generally a contract will be for 12 to 24 months. Most contracts will provide the employer and the employee with some sort of early cancellation rights. For instance, a contract may state that either party can cancel the contract without cause simply by providing 30 to 60 days' notice of the intent to do so. Other contracts may allow the employer unilaterally to cancel the contract for just cause, usually the employee's failure to perform duties diligently. Just cause also could cancel the contract in case a physician commits a felony or loses the medical license. The term section of a contract also may discuss when you will become eligible to become a shareholder. Typically this section discusses intent (if all goes well) but it is not binding. This is another reason to know with whom you are practicing. The promise of becoming a shareholder and the reality of becoming a shareholder depend on the integrity of the physicians who hired you. From the onset, you should discuss in general terms the details of becoming an owner of the practice.
- *Duties of employee:* This paragraph will outline the professional services expected of you. It will define the employee/employer relationship and probably will require that you devote all your professional time and attention to practicing medicine for the employer. In other words, no moonlighting. If you want to teach or do research, negotiate this issue now, and make sure that the contract specifies exactly what will be expected of you to avoid any future misunderstandings. This section also may outline your responsibilities in taking calls.
- *Salary and benefits:* Pay close attention to this section of the contract. Of course, this section will outline your base salary and any incentive bonuses. It should also discuss the following benefits:
    1. Vacation time (typically two to four weeks)
    2. Time for continuing medical education (typically one to two weeks with an allowance of $2,000 to $3,000, paid by the employer, toward your continuing medical education costs)
    3. Sick leave (typically two to three weeks)
    4. Pension plan eligibility (typically eligible after one year)
    5. Malpractice insurance premiums (typically paid by employer; do not forget to discuss who will pay for a tail policy if you leave the practice)

6. Disability insurance coverage
7. Group term life insurance coverage
8. Health insurance coverage for you and your family
9. Medical reimbursement plan
10. Auto expense reimbursement
11. Professional dues and subscriptions
12. Business entertainment allowance
13. Moving expenses.

Benefit packages vary widely depending on your specialty and the group you are joining. A knowledgeable advisor can give you a realistic idea of what you should expect.

- *Disability or incapacity of employee:* The contract should address in some detail what will happen in case you are disabled. Generally, contracts provide for some form of salary continuation by the employer until your disability insurance benefits begin to pay.
- *Death benefit:* Again, the contract should address what happens in the event of your death during the term of the contract.
- *Medical records:* Contracts usually state that medical records or charts are the property of the employer and will not be turned over to the employee unless a patient specifically requests the transfer.
- *Covenant not to compete:* Most contracts restrict your ability to compete with your employer should you leave the practice. Typically, these covenants not to compete will restrain you from opening an office within a certain distance of your former employer for a stated period of time after you leave.
- *Other issues:* Other clauses that you can expect to find in physician employment contracts are the following:
  1. a clause that requires binding arbitration (as opposed to litigation) should any disputes arise from the contract
  2. a requirement that you become board-certified within a reasonable period of time
  3. a confidentiality clause
  4. discussions regarding policies and procedures specific to the group of which you need to be aware
  5. discussions regarding severance pay, if any.

Final Words

It is not within the scope of this lesson to discuss in detail the elements of buying into or out of an existing practice. Because it is a related topic, however, two words are in order: Be careful.

One of the ironies of medical practices is that, although they typically provide good incomes for physicians, the practices themselves do not have a lot of value. This is because the only assets that practices have are usually medical equipment, which rapidly loses its value, and accounts receivable. The accounts receivable are the direct result of the work of the present owner and may or may not continue if you buy the practice. For example, an experienced plastic surgeon may have a large patient base due to years of experience and a fine reputation. If you were to buy this practice, however, you might find that the patient base sees you as new and inexperienced. The flow of patients may go to another, more senior plastic surgeon in the area. You have now paid a premium for a practice and are, in reality, starting from scratch to build it.

The same general philosophy holds true for buying into a group in which you have been an employee. Your buy-in should consist primarily of your hard work and the profit the group made from it during your initial years as a non-owner employee. After two to five years, you should be allowed to become an owner in the practice. The cost of ownership should be based on a reasonable formula. Examples range from no buy-in cost to you to a buy-in based on the corporation's net book value plus the discounted value of accounts receivable. Generally, the longer you are a non-partner employee, the lower your ultimate buy-in will be. Again, buy-ins are complex, and you should seek the advice of experienced professionals.

One final related issue is taking a salaried position with a managed care group. In general, most of the contract provisions covered above also apply to managed care contracts. You can expect salaries to be somewhat lower and benefits potentially better, however, over a longer period of time. Managed care groups like to put golden handcuffs on physicians by means of excellent long-term benefits packages.

Currently, the managed care business is rapidly changing, and compensation packages to physician employees vary significantly. The best advice is to get advice from a competent, experienced professional.

◆ Chapter 9 ◆

Lagniappe

Lagniappe (lan yap′): A small present given to a customer or client.

LESSON 9–1: COMPUTERIZE

Technology sprints by us in a blur of megabytes, RAMs, faxes, and laser-powered communication tools. Every day, office technology becomes more sophisticated and less expensive. Most of us who are 40-something or more, however, still gaze upon computers with awe and fear.

Nonetheless, my advice to you is to computerize your office. You would never dream of ignoring the information that a computed tomographic scanner, magnetic resonance imager, or other piece of high-tech equipment could provide in critical cases. The medical office of the future will have to adopt that same attitude toward equipping itself.

> **◆ MEDICAL PRACTICE MANAGEMENT TRUTH 11 ◆**
>
> **Competition will demand that your office keep up with technology.**

Hardware and software costs for installing a first-class computer system for a small medical practice are $5,000 to $10,000. Naturally the cost increases for larger offices, but not dramatically. The expense of computerization often is recouped in the first year of operation by means of:

- speedier, more accurate filing of insurance claims forms
- quicker collection of accounts receivable and quicker recognition of and action taken on past due accounts
- reduced employee costs for paperwork preparation
- more efficient patient scheduling

Here are some office computerization tips:

- There are several excellent medical office manager software systems that perform patient scheduling, insurance claims forms preparation (including electronic filing), and charges and collections recording. Have your office manager meet with several software companies and test their products thoroughly before you decide which package to purchase. Ask the software vendor for the names of several physicians, preferably of your specialty, who are currently using the software. Call them to see how satisfied they are with the software and with the vendor's support and training programs. Don't be afraid to engage the services of a competent expert to help you select the system that is best for you. Ask other physicians or medical contacts who have already computerized for references. You might also check with the physician services departments of local hospitals because they often keep a list of available computer consultants. Also, your CPA may be able to help you. Your consultant should aid you in the following:
  1. Selecting a vendor:
     —How many installations does the vendor currently have?
     —How many support personnel does the vendor have?
     —How many years has the vendor been in existence?
  2. Selecting hardware:
     —speed
     —language
     —purchase price
     —five-year maintenance cost
     —installation cost
     —maintenance response time
  3. Selecting software:
     —user friendly
     —special features that you may need

—updates
—purchase cost
—five-year maintenance cost
—conversion cost
—exact programs that you will need

4. Arranging for installation
5. Arranging for staff training and ongoing support.

- Buy clone hardware. Several companies sell first-class IBM-compatible hardware at reasonable prices. Companies such as 47th Street Photo [(800) 221-7774] and Gateway 2000 [(800) 523-2000] offer excellent state-of-the-art hardware at competitive prices.
- Many medical office manager software packages do not offer accounts payable and payroll functions. The good news is that there is a program call *Quicken* by Intuit [(800) 624-8742] that provides both these programs for about $75. Our firm uses *Quicken* for accounts payable, tracking receipts, reconciling the bank statement, and preparing rudimentary in-house financial statements. I can unequivocally tell you that it is the best software value on the market today.
- Expect some frustration and staff resistance for the first 90 days of computerization. Encourage your staff to master the computer. Within a year, they will wonder how they ever managed without it.

LESSON 9–2: TO INCORPORATE OR NOT TO INCORPORATE

Physicians often ask, "Does it still make sense for physicians to incorporate their practices?" Absolutely. In fact, I would not practice under any other legal form. Here's why:

- Advantages of incorporating:
  1. *Limited liability:* Although a professional corporation cannot shield you from your acts of malpractice, it may, in most states, provide a substantial degree of limited liability that is unavailable to solo practitioners or partnerships. See your attorney for an in-depth explanation of how a professional corporation shields your assets. In today's litigious atmosphere, this advantage alone may be reason enough to incorporate.
  2. *Fringe benefits:* Corporations enjoy favorable tax treatment for certain fringe benefits that are unavailable to solo practitioners and partnerships. These benefits include the before-tax deductibility of disability insurance, health insurance, certain medical expenses via a medical reimbursement plan, and limited amounts of group term life insurance.
  3. *Continuity of life:* A corporation continues indefinitely even after the death of a shareholder.
  4. *Likelihood of audit:* It has been my experience that professional corporations are audited less frequently by the Internal Revenue Service than solo practitioners, who report their income and expenses on schedule C.
- Disadvantages of incorporating:
  1. *Additional recordkeeping:* Corporate income tax returns need to be prepared annually. This additional expense is far outweighed by the advantages of incorporating, however.
  2. *Year-end tax planning:* Professional corporations are conduits. This means that year-end tax planning is important to avoid double taxation. Competent advisors will ensure that you avoid double taxation.

LESSON 9–3: SOURCES

The following is a list of journals, magazines, books, and organizations for the physician who wants to know more about the business of medicine and/or his or her personal finances. Each publication or organization is excellent, and the cost of subscribing or joining will be repaid to you many times over by what you learn and apply from each.

- Journals and magazines
  1. *Medical Economics* [(800) 621-4431]
  2. *Medical Economics for Surgeons* [(800) 621-4431]
  3. *Physician's Advisory* [(215) 828-3888]
  4. *Consumer Reports* [(800) 766-9988]
  5. *Money* [(800) 633-9970]
  6. *Smart Money* [(800) 444-4204]
  7. *Forbes* [(800) 888-9896]
  8. *Physician's Management* [(218) 723-9200]
  9. *Medical Office Manager* [(617) 639-1872]
  10. *Kiplinger's Personal Finance* [(800) 544-0155]
- General books on business management
  1. *Swim with the Sharks*, by Harvey MacKay
  2. *How To Win Friends and Influence People*, by Dale Carnegie
  3. *Marketing Your Clinical Practice*, by Neil Baum, MD
  4. *How To Win Customers and Keep Them for Life*, by Michael LeBoeuf
- Organizations
  1. The Medical Group Management Association [(303) 753-1111]
  2. The American Hospital Association [(202) 638-1100]

LESSON 9–4: THE MEDICAL PRACTICE MANAGEMENT TRUTHS

1. To enjoy future financial success, physicians must understand more than practicing medicine. They must understand the business of medicine.
2. Ultimately, all your business and personal financial concerns will fall into one of three areas:
   - your medical practice
   - your retirement plan
   - your personal financial situation.
3. Without a doubt, your single most important practice management tool is properly prepared and analyzed financial statements.
4. Never mold your practice around a problem. The best run practices are those that make the tough decisions.
5. A medical practice's fee setting strategy is an integral part of practice management.
6. Physicians must understand and accept three realities to come to terms with managed care:
   - Medicine is now big business.
   - The driving force behind managed care is profit.
   - Providers who learn to negotiate with managed care companies will fare best.
7. No one will ever be as concerned about your money as you.
8. Competition is going to force marketing onto the practice of medicine.
9. The most valuable asset in your practice is your employees.
10. In most cases, your ability or inability to retire will be directly related to how much you have accumulated in your pension plan.
11. Competition will demand that your office keep up with technology.
12. At some point in your career, time will become more important than money.

◆ Epilog ◆

Monopoly

> ◆ **MEDICAL PRACTICE MANAGEMENT TRUTH 12** ◆
>
> **At some point in your career, time will become more important than money.**

Dr. James Dobson, host of the radio show "Focus on the Family," is one of the people whom I respect most in this world. He tells a story of an event in his life that is almost identical to my own experience.

My wife's family loves to get together and play board games. They eat, talk, and enjoy one another while not really paying much attention to the game at hand. I can't stand it. But one night they pulled out my game: *Monopoly*.

Now this was a game I could sink my teeth into. This was real life. I played intensely, buying property and houses as fast as I could. My houses were replaced by hotels, and soon I controlled most of the board. The first person I forced out of the game was my wife's 78-year-old grandmother. She never stood a chance. I was ruthless. One by one I picked off the other players, until each of them was thoroughly mad at me. Finally, they all quit and left me alone to clean up the pieces.

As I sat there with my empty victory, it came to me: It all goes back into the box at the end of the game. All the cash, the property, the buildings, everything we own goes back into the box. Then someone else comes along to play the game.

In the end, it is our relationships with our friends and family and our God that counts. The game will go on without us.

Postscript

In this book, I have given you the best ideas that I have for solving many of the major problems that physicians confront in the management of their practices. I would love to hear about methods that you have used to tackle tough management problems. Please write and tell me the best, worst, most useful, and funniest ideas you have used in your practice. Also, if you have any questions or comments about this book, please contact me:

Robert W. Katz
1515 Poydras Street, Suite 1800
New Orleans, LA 70112
(504) 525-8524

INSERT

TAB

Index

C

D

E

F

G

H

I

9 780834 205321

Printed in Dunstable, United Kingdom

88190713R00112